Praise for *L̲*

"A well-considered prescription for th̲ first-person stories and interviews wit̲ human case for national reform. A sup̲ ....cing with their parents' final days and anxiou̲ ....ore control over their own rites of passage, as well as for health professionals who need to hear this story from the other side." —*Kirkus Reviews* (starred review)

"Most people find it difficult to face their own mortality and that of their loved ones. This book compassionately and skillfully addresses this difficult emotional issue. This well-written and thoughtful book, filled with surveys, interviews, and personal stories, is highly recommended." —*Library Journal*

"Stephen Kiernan's message is one for all of us who will face the prospect of caring for a dying family member or friend. *Last Rights* is a compelling examination." —Donald Schumacher, president, National Hospice and Palliative Care Organization

"*Last Rights* paints a frightening picture of the disorganized, deficient, and disastrous ways many people are cared for and die. Thankfully, Kiernan goes beyond exposé to uncover hopeful progress and practical ways to protect and nurture the people we love." —Ira Byock, M.D., professor of Palliative Medicine, Dartmouth Medical School, author of *Dying Well* and *The Four Things That Matter Most*

"Damn, I wish I'd had this book before my own father died. Part a guide to thinking through the policy questions surrounding the end of life, and part an informal handbook for helping with the deaths of your own loved ones, it also offers a final and supreme gift: the chance to begin thinking about what your own life means in the context of its inevitable end." —Bill McKibben, author of *The End of Nature*

"With an uncommon mix of stories and scholarship Stephen Kiernan has described the challenges that remain at life's end, despite efforts to reform care over the past few decades. With candor, clarity, and an advocate's sense of urgency, he seeks to understand why our acute care system has been so resistant to change and how we can infuse greater humanity to life's final chapter." —Joseph J. Fins, M.D., F.A.C.P., Chief of the Division of Medical Ethics, Weill Medical College of Cornell University, and author of *A Palliative Ethic of Care: Clinical Wisdom at Life's End*

"With the heart of a poet and the skill of an investigative reporter, Mr. Kiernan has written a powerful examination of end-of-life care. . . . Mr. Kiernan's book is a powerful reminder of the ongoing need for reform in the way our institutions relate to the dying and their families. It serves as a wake-up call. . . . Kiernan is unafraid to write of mystery, comfort, and compassion." —Linda F. Piotrowski, MTS, NACC Cert., in *Vision,* the publication of the National Association of Catholic Chaplains

"It is simply human nature that no matter how often we have dealt with death, we are never prepared for it. *Last Rights* offers practical advice and, surprisingly, optimism." —Reese Vaughn, "Books at the Crossroads," *The Victoria Advocate*

"In *Last Rights* Kiernan offers suggestions to the government, to the medical profession, and to the American public—suggestions that could change the course of many patients from the prospect of a technological death to a better way. His investigative insight combined with an ability to tell a gripping story make this book a must-read." —*Burlington Free Press*

"*Last Rights* employs a three-pronged strategy. It defines how the end of life has changed in this country and presents the options available to families caring for a loved one. Second, it describes the barriers to providing a dignified final chapter in life, and finally, it includes many stories of families who have accomplished a beautiful end-of-life experience." —*The Charlotte News*

"As aging baby boomers become ever more involved in the deaths of parents and friends, they will press for changes in laws and the medical system. . . . Terminally ill people must push hard if they want to maintain control of the end of their lives and die with dignity, Kiernan found." —*Daily News*

"Wise words, and timely for everyone in the healing professions, anyone active in church or charity work, and all who may become the primary caregiver for an ill or elderly friend or relative." —hop's log, John Hopkins Miami, Florida

LAST RIGHTS

RESCUING THE END OF LIFE FROM
THE MEDICAL SYSTEM

STEPHEN P. KIERNAN

 ST. MARTIN'S GRIFFIN ☂ NEW YORK

The stories of Colin Murray Parkes, M.D., and Balfour Mount, M.D. (pages 90–91) come from the film *Pioneers of Hospice: Changing the Face of Dying*. Their reflections appear with the permission of Madison-Deane Initiative, which produced the film.

The Journal of Palliative Medicine granted permission for two items: medical students' reactions after a first exposure to hospice care (pages 98–101), and David Weissman, M.D.'s personal essay about doctors' desire to control the dying process (page 187).

The exchange of letters entitled "Crying in Stairwells" (pages 117–118) appears with the permission of the *Journal of the American Medical Association*, Sept. 7, 1994, vol. 272, no. 9, p. 659, copyright © American Medical Association. All rights reserved.

The selection from Chuang-Tzu (page 221) appears with the permission of the translator, David Hinton.

Discussion of the hospice at the Louisiana State Penitentiary comes from the Open Society Institute documentary *Angola Prison Hospice: Opening the Door* copyright © 1998 Open Society Institute. All rights reserved. Used by permission.

www.stmartins.com

Book design by Gretchen Achilles

Library of Congress Cataloging-in-Publication Data

Kiernan, Stephen.
    Last rights : rescuing the end of life from the medical system / Stephen Kiernan.
        p. cm.
    Includes bibliographical references.
    ISBN-13: 978-0-312-37464-8
    ISBN-10: 0-312-37464-X
    1. Terminal care. 2. Death. I. Title.

R726.8.K52 2006
179.7—dc22

2006047449

First St. Martin's Griffin Edition: December 2007

10 9 8 7 6 5 4 3 2 1

To the six people I most admire on this earth,
my brothers and sisters

CONTENTS

INTRODUCTION

I n the early morning of August 12, 2002, Arlene Charron of Lyndonville, Vermont, lay struggling for breath.

She was eighty-five years old. She had been sick with respiratory
illness for months. Well before she entered Northeastern Vermont Regional Hospital in St. Johnsbury, Arlene had written legal instructions not
to be kept alive by a ventilator. Yet in the final days of her life, she was attached to a machine, anyway. To prevent her reflexively yanking out the
tube that snaked down her throat into her lungs, Arlene's arms had to be
strapped down or she had to be sedated into motionlessness, or both.

Arlene's physician was Dr. Lloyd "Tim" Thompson, who'd been treating her for more than twenty years. Although he practiced in a remote
corner of a rural state, Thompson was no small-town quack. Educated at
Yale and the University of Pennsylvania, the newly trained doctor had
come to Lyndonville in 1973, as part of a federal program that exempted
physicians from the draft if they agreed to practice in an underserved rural area for several years. After the Vietnam War ended, however, Thompson stayed. His tiny clinic grew into a seven-thousand-square-foot
regional health service allied with the prestigious Dartmouth-Hitchcock
Medical Center in New Hampshire.

Over the decades Thompson rose in the medical community until he
was president of the hospital's medical staff and medical director of a local nursing home. He even became president of the Vermont Medical Society, the statewide association of doctors. He wore half-glasses low on his
nose and dressed in corduroys and button-down shirts with the sleeves
rolled up. He met regularly with the governor.

Thompson had deep roots in the community he served, after thirty
years of house calls and office appointments. In Lyndonville and the surrounding hill towns, almost everybody knew who "Dr. Tim" was.

Most important, Thompson was considered expert in end-of-life care. He had founded the county hospice, which provides medical and emotional care at home for people who are dying, and chaired a statewide committee to improve treatment of the terminally ill. By training, experience, and inclination, this physician was ideally suited to help Arlene Charron.

She was not unfamiliar with death, either. She had been predeceased by two brothers, two sisters, and two daughters. Her husband, Nelson, had died at home, in Thompson's care, in November 2000. That year Arlene signed a durable power of attorney for health care, a legal document directing what care she wanted to receive should she become unable to express those wishes herself. The document said that if she became terminally ill, she wanted "only care directed to my comfort and dignity" and did not want care "the primary purpose of which is to prolong my life."

By the summer of 2002 Arlene suffered from lung disease, severe chronic obstructive pulmonary disease, and lung lesions. There was no hope for a cure. But neither was there an expectation that her lungs would suddenly fail, which happened in early August in the hospital. Rather than let her die, the physician in charge of her care in Thompson's absence put her on a ventilator. Why this doctor acted contrary to her instructions remains unknown; he may simply have been unaware of them. Besides, doctors routinely ignore or overrule patients' care directives. The next day Thompson sought to honor Arlene's wishes by removing her from the machine. She became so agitated, though, that he immediately reinserted the breathing tube.

Normally a person who does not want to be kept alive by a ventilator receives morphine, to quell the sense of suffocation as breathing assistance is gradually removed. If the patient suffers, the dosage is increased. There is an art to performing this process compassionately, doctors say; many watch the patient's brow and add morphine whenever it furrows. Eventually the patient is pain-free and machine-free. Death may then come over a span of hours or days. Among medical ethicists this approach is not considered killing a patient, because the physician treats a patient's genuine distress while letting nature take whatever course it may. In rare cases the patient actually recovers.

Over the next few days Thompson tried repeatedly to wean Arlene from the machine, without success. Her family witnessed these struggles. Each time she was put back on a machine she did not want. What happened next is alleged in later state physician regulators' documents.

On August 12 at 8:30 A.M., Thompson began the process of removing the breathing tube once again. He gave Arlene a 5-milligram dose of Versed, a sedative that relieves the anxiety of people struggling to breathe. He also gave her 20 milligrams of morphine for pain. At 8:36 he gave Arlene another dose of both drugs. That was a telltale decision, because morphine requires ten minutes to take effect. Did he want to stay ahead of any signs of discomfort? Or was he out of his depth? The public record does not reveal his intentions.

At 8:40 he gave her another 10 milligrams of morphine, and at 8:45 another dose of Versed. That action said even more: administering such large doses so rapidly could reduce the body's initiative to breathe. Instead of letting nature take its course, there was a strong risk that nature could be pushed. Certainly there was no evidence of the fine art of pain management.

At 8:45 Thompson removed the ventilator tube, after which he gave another 10 milligrams of Versed and 20 milligrams of morphine. A perfectly healthy person receiving that much medication would have a reduced capacity to breathe. Arlene might as well have been a hundred feet underwater.

Once she was free of the machine, her breathing rate dropped sharply, as one might expect. But then Thompson did something extraordinary. He gave Arlene 10 milligrams of Norcuron. That drug is not made for end-of-life care. It does not block pain. It has no sedative effect. Norcuron's purpose is to cause paralysis. It is designed for patients in surgery, to prevent them from shifting or interfering with life-sustaining feeding or breathing tubes. Government-approved guidelines stipulate that Norcuron is to be used only on patients connected to a ventilator. A perfectly healthy person receiving 10 milligrams of Norcuron would collapse, stop breathing, and die.

For Arlene, the dose made her incapable of showing any distress she may have felt. Panic would be concealed, her brow smooth throughout. An expressionless state may have comforted her family and physician, but it meant that no one could know the character of her life's final experiences—whether calm and pain-free or paralyzed and terrified. Within minutes of the Norcuron injection, Arlene Charron was dead.

A clinician in the room understood immediately what had happened. This nurse or technician's name has never become public, but he or she went directly to the hospital's chief executive officer, Paul Bengston.

"A review of the situation began in like seconds," Bengston said. That inquiry consisted of a "peer review," an oversight system in which physicians evaluate one another's work. The confidentiality of peer reviews is protected by law in the reasonable hope that doctors—free of fear of a malpractice suit over an error—will reveal mistakes to their colleagues and thereby learn how to prevent repeating them. It is illegal for doctors to disclose what they have heard in a fellow physician's peer review. And it is extremely rare for the content of a peer review to escape the sacrosanct walls of the hospital.

Yet on August 20 Thompson's hospital filed a complaint against him with the Medical Practice Board, the state agency that regulates doctors.

That is where I came in.

For the previous two years I had written extensively about that board in my work as an investigative reporter at the *Burlington Free Press*. For a modest-size daily in a small state, the *Free Press* in that era was a scrappy newspaper. After an eight-month investigation, we had revealed serious flaws in the state's oversight of physicians. We found an orthopedic surgeon whose history included nine lawsuits, operations on wrong body parts, and allegations of errors that left patients maimed and in two cases dead. Yet regulators allowed him to continue to practice medicine. The small hospital where he performed surgery (and generated one-third of inpatient revenue) continued to employ him. Worst, state law shielded the doctor's record almost entirely from the public.

State legislators vowed to pass reforms to make regulators tougher on doctors and to reveal more of doctors' histories to the public. The fate of those bills was uncertain, however; lobbyists had defeated similar proposals three times in the past decade.

So we piled on. We revealed a surgeon whose errors resulted in amputations and death. We exposed a doctor who over six years wrote herself prescriptions for eighteen thousand doses of the narcotic Percocet. We proved that a disproportionate share of sanctioned physicians worked at one small hospital. We reported that psychiatrists were disciplined more than any other specialty, because of inappropriate sexual relations with patients. And in all these cases, the public did not know.

The bill passed in the House with only two votes against. The Senate vote was unanimous. For the signing ceremony, Governor Howard Dean—himself a physician—invited people whose tragedies our stories had told.

It was all old-fashioned, shoe-leather reporting: late hours and long drives, arguments with editors and threats from doctors' lawyers, wading through court records and reassuring a publisher who was unafraid of telling the truth but equally uninterested in getting sued.

Professionally, in other words, it was all enormous fun. And now, only five months later, Arlene Charron's case could test the reform law down to its bones. That the physician in question was politically powerful only raised the stakes. I cleared my desk and prepared for the fireworks.

They never came. The Medical Practice Board released a document declaring that it was aware of the incident, understood the ethical issues the case raised, and would conduct a period of reflection and investigation.

Then hospital CEO Bengston announced that Thompson would continue as head of the medical staff. "Dr. Thompson is an outstanding physician," he said. "I have every confidence in the quality of the work that he does."

Thompson's three partners in the medical clinic stood by him, too. The Vermont Medical Society kept him on as president. "We feel it would be unfair to prejudge Dr. Thompson in advance of the Medical Practice Board rendering its opinion," said executive vice president Paul Harrington.

The medical community was not alone. The case came before Vermont attorney general William Sorrell, a former criminal prosecutor who built his reputation by solving decades-old murder cases. If the allegations were accurate, Sorrell speculated that the facts in a case like this could result in voluntary manslaughter charges, a felony bringing a fifteen-year jail sentence. Yet Sorrell said he would not file charges for some time, if ever.

I was beyond perplexed. The case seemed simple. A physician, however seemingly able, had crossed a clear ethical and legal line. There had to be consequences, or it would give tacit permission to other doctors to do the same. The state's Roman Catholic bishop, Kenneth Angell, denounced Thompson's actions: "God is the author of life and only God may decide when a life shall end." But the bishop was a lone voice.

I drove to Lyndonville. I dug through public records and obtained the death certificate. Arlene Charron had been pronounced dead at 9:12 A.M., August 12, 2002. Dr. Thompson signed her certificate. In the portion labeled "manner of death," he checked the box that read "natural."

Arlene's family declined to be interviewed, so I spoke with her friends. They weren't upset. I interviewed the parish priest, who knew her, visited her home, and performed her funeral service. His bishop notwithstanding, the priest was not exercised about what had happened. I drove by Arlene's house, a small Cape on Pinehurst Street. A neighbor was out getting the mail. Eighty-three-year-old John Gray invited me in.

The entry was cluttered with clothes, boots, stacks of newspaper, and an oxygen tank. A clear tube led from the tank into the living room.

"I have emphysema, diabetes, and what is that other thing," said John's wife, Jeanette, age eighty-one, as she sniffed from the tube under her nose. She and John had been Arlene's neighbors for forty years. One of their daughters had married one of Arlene's sons. Jeanette was also a fan of Dr. Thompson.

"He's still my doctor and will stay my doctor," she said, squinting at my legal pad as I took notes. "I go to him for good care and straight talk."

She did not want to see Thompson disciplined for what had happened. "When my time comes, I want to be able to still go to him."

Later that day, after weeks of leaving unreturned messages at Dr. Thompson's office, I caught him at home. He said his lawyers had given him strict instructions not to speak with anyone, especially me. That is the kind of statement a reporter routinely ignores. I started my interview, asking if he could explain the puzzle I had found. There was a long pause.

"Before we can even begin to discuss this, you need to do some reading," he said. He immediately rattled off a dozen articles in medical journals, by physician-researchers such as Timothy Quill, M.D., Andrew Billings, M.D., and Sherwin Nuland, M.D., experts in the care of people who are dying. "I might answer your questions—I might—once you've done your homework."

Soon I tracked down those articles, in such publications as the *Journal of the American Medical Association,* the *New England Journal of Medicine,* and the *Journal of Palliative Medicine.* Instead of providing a solution to my puzzle, these research papers offered evidence that it was more complex than I had realized. Arlene Charron's struggles—and her family's and her physician's—reflected similar difficulties all across the country. That discovery led me to many more questions, to dozens of books and medical journal articles, to hundreds of interviews, even to frank contemplation of my own death.

It was no longer old-fashioned reporting. When you interview a dying woman in what turns out to be her last lucid conversation, when you stand beside family members weeping over their father's death, when you accompany a woman from final diagnosis to cemetery, you simply cannot maintain traditional journalistic objectivity. You become involved, you care, you mourn.

Fortunately, when you see people die well, their family uplifted by the opportunity to demonstrate love through diligent caretaking under hard circumstances, you can also celebrate the unique joys that are possible at the end of life.

I also spent time with many physicians and researchers, and came to almost contradictory conclusions about them. On the plus side, each of the doctors I interviewed—every one—was impeccably educated, master of a vast volume of knowledge, and sincerely motivated to help people. These physicians battled with medical and insurance bureaucracies and persisted despite the ever present cloud of possible lawsuits. On the minus side, however, they too often revealed themselves as unequipped to help the dying and strangely untrained in something all of their patients were certain to experience.

All that research led me to an inescapable conclusion: the manner in which Americans die has changed. It used to be sudden, and now it is gradual. It used to happen at home, and now it occurs primarily in hospitals and nursing homes.

I also learned that health-care institutions are not prepared for this shift. I learned that families are facing painful questions about when to continue medical treatment and when to say enough. I learned that patients who try to exert some control over their final days often encounter a medical culture indifferent to their values and desires.

These lessons may sound like a set of depressing problems, but they are only part of the story. I also found times when things had gone right, and these stories were uplifting, moving, even inspirational.

With some hesitation I told friends what I was learning, and thereby made another discovery: if I mentioned my research even superficially, people invariably replied by describing deaths they had witnessed or loved ones they had lost. Their eagerness to tell these stories, their near compulsion to recount some of their lives' deepest experiences, was unlike anything I had encountered before. I started writing the stories down.

Without realizing it, I had begun work on this book.

Part One describes how dying in America has changed in the past thirty years. We used to die primarily of heart attacks, strokes, and accidents. Now we die mostly of cancer, Alzheimer's, and AIDS. That shift presents an opportunity for sublime end-of-life experiences—last wishes fulfilled, pain managed, relationships repaired, spiritual calm attained—which almost everyone misses.

Next I felt an imperative to demystify gradual dying, to discuss its stages in unvarnished fashion. That's Part Two. The idea was not to minimize the loss people feel when someone they love dies. Rather, the intent is to help people understand how dying typically takes place today. We cannot so easily fear something we have begun to know.

The next three parts have a similar structure, as each investigates a subset of the people challenged by gradual dying. Part Three tells the stories of physicians who, however great their skills, have found themselves untrained in end-of-life care and unequipped to help patients die with dignity. This section also offers success stories of physicians who have found unequalled personal and professional satisfaction in caring for patients near the end of their lives.

Part Four looks at families and the weighty decisions they must now make about their loved ones' care. It investigates some of the challenges, then highlights families who have done an outstanding job in caring for their parents and siblings and spouses. These families demonstrate a new kind of love—vulnerable, courageous, enduring.

Part Five chronicles the predicaments of patients themselves, who know their end is approaching and who must summon the bravery to face mortality—and thereby maximize the quality of their remaining days. When that effort goes awry, the stories can be heartbreaking. But in some cases, terminally ill people describe last wishes beautifully answered, lives that end literally with singing and dancing. These people represent the potential, the peaceful future every American deserves.

Lest the challenges of obtaining good end-of-life care seem too daunting, it's important to note that even people utterly unschooled in this work can learn. Part Six makes this point by telling the story of my parents, both of whom presented doctors and our family with difficult caretaking decisions. My father received every possible medical intervention, at great expense and with negligible result. Five years later my mother died at home in her bed, her pain managed and family at her side. What my siblings and I learned, our society must learn. If we could do it, so can you.

The task of providing an excellent end-of-life experience will be vastly simpler, though, if the health-care system adapts to the reality of gradual dying. Part Seven offers two approaches. The first is somewhat hard-boiled—an agenda for improvements in everything from physician training to consumer activism to Medicare rules to patients' rights. There are concrete steps that government, the medical community, and the American public can take to reckon with a reality that is grim today but does not have to be so in the future.

The second approach is more emotional and personal. I mentioned earlier that the endeavor of this book required a departure from journalistic norms. In addition to objective research, I also received powerful instruction from people who were dying, their families, and their medical caregivers. Beyond the policy ideas, therefore, Part Seven contains some of those lessons. They are not about death. Their ultimate message is about life, its preciousness, and the importance of living meaningfully each day.

TO TELL STORIES EFFICIENTLY, this book uses two kinds of shorthand. One is the word *families*. Naturally that refers to a person's blood relations. But given the way people can gather near at the end of a person's life, the word is also meant in a broader sense, to include the neighbors, friends, work associates, and others who may participate in the caretaking.

The other shorthand is the word *doctors*. Again my intent is to imply a larger meaning, invoking not only physicians but also the complex systems in which they work: networks of hospital and nursing-home administrators, health insurers, medical educators, researchers, regulators, and more. This book finds fault with a few doctors, granted, but I'm convinced that most physicians care deeply about their work and their patients. Part Three relates the frustrations that many well-meaning doctors experience when trying to do a good job for people who are dying. Broader blame and greater imperative to change falls upon those unresponsive health-care systems.

It is probably worth declaring a few things that this book is not going to cover in much depth. Foremost among these is cultural differences in attitudes toward dying. The American populace is simply too diverse for anything but a superficial treatment of the ways that various religions and nationalities treat such issues as receiving blood transfusions, donating organs for transplant, touching a dead body, and so on. There are many degrees of taboo around death, but none counters the imperative to help people make the most of their last days.

This book is also not going to delve deeply into physician-assisted suicide, near-death experiences, life after death, or coping with grief. Though undoubtedly interesting and important, these topics were to my mind less urgent than the questions of how to help our loved ones die in peace and how to attain such an end for ourselves. The focus of this book's enterprise is not death and its aftermath, but life, how its waning days could be peaceful and pain-free, and how caring for people at their most vulnerable can be an incredibly fulfilling experience.

• • •

EVENTUALLY VERMONT'S MEDICAL PRACTICE BOARD did issue a decision on Dr. Thompson. He received the lightest disciplinary action the board can render, a reprimand. The allegations against him were never proven, because the case resolved without a public hearing, but Thompson signed a state document in which he did not contest that he gave the patient Norcuron. The board's ruling included a detailed description of the kind of end-of-life care Vermonters deserve, with the clear implication that Thompson had not met that standard. His sanction was widely seen as symbolic only, a slap on the wrist. Then the attorney general announced that he was not going to prosecute the doctor for manslaughter. "The patient's family knew what he was doing," Sorrell said. "They were supportive."

Case closed. To his credit, Sorrell went on to form a task force of physicians, nurses, hospice leaders, and others to improve end-of-life care in Vermont. Their work led to a new law strengthening advance directives, so that in the future people in Arlene Charron's predicament will be less likely to wind up on machines they do not desire.

Thompson resigned as president of the medical society, issuing a public apology but remaining a leader in the organization. He still practices medicine in Vermont's remote Northeast Kingdom.

In late 2004 the county probate court issued an order for Arlene's death certificate to be changed. The manner of death no longer reads "natural." In an apt expression of how ambiguous officials found the case, the manner is forevermore recorded as "undetermined."

Arlene Charron was buried in the small cemetery east of Lyndonville, across the road from the Little League diamond. She is survived by seven children, twenty-three grandchildren, twenty-four great-grandchildren, and two great-great-grandchildren. She is also outlived by the larger story about dramatic changes in dying in America and how society's response is tragically lagging—a problem in which her ignored instructions, her family's anguish, her physician's error, and her struggling last breaths are unfortunately typical.

PART ONE

THE IMPRINT
A BODY MAKES

*Even in the valley of the shadow of death,
two and two do not make six.*
—LEO TOLSTOY

CHAPTER ONE

LAST HOURS

On the final night of his life, Jack happened to glance out the window just before eleven and notice that it was snowing: fat flakes cascading past the porch light, changing direction in a puff of wind like a school of fish veering from a predator.

Had Jack known what lay ahead, the seven hours left to him, he might have done something other than turn back to the television. He might have reached for the phone and called his daughter, a college freshman, to send her his love and let her tap him for spending money one last time. He might have climbed the stairs to his son's room, interrupting that bookish boy's latest fascination for a discussion of how to help his mother weather widowhood. Jack might have gone to his wife, already in bed, to plan for life without him or remind her where his will was stored or revisit their fondest memories like jewelers scrutinizing rubies. He might simply have decided to go to the window, to watch the snow and contemplate the infinite.

Instead, Jack plunged his hand into a bag of potato chips, washed a mouthful down with the warm dregs of a beer, and watched the Celtics lose in overtime. He lit a cigarette, an unfiltered Camel—he reasoned that if you're going to smoke, you might as well taste it. Though he'd never seen the Celtics play in person, in the morning his loyalty would cost him both five bucks and a razzing from Bo, a coworker buddy who favored the Lakers.

It was December 1, 1976, a Monday, and too early for snow. Jack switched off the TV, crushed out his smoke. With a beefy forearm he gathered the empties against his stomach and shuffled into the kitchen.

After shoving everything into the trash, Jack went back through the house dousing lights. He moved slowly, aware that lately the furniture crowded him because he'd put on so much weight. Always a hefty guy, Jack now had a bona fide belly, a smoker's cough he hacked through some mornings, a general sluggishness in his blood. He would have gone to a doctor, but why bother when you already know what the problem is? You're getting older, fifty-six in April, and the beer and the sweet tooth and the butts and the lack of exercise have a bigger effect now than when you were twenty-six. Jack put a hand on his lower back as he bent down to turn off a table lamp. Yes, he should cut down. And exercise. Definitely quit the Camels, God forbid. But a man cannot be disciplined about everything. A man who has worked hard all his life also deserves some pleasures, doesn't he?

This line of thinking was so familiar that it was nearly furniture, too. Room by room, Jack flicked switches and left darkness behind him. At the top of the stairs he paused, dimly aware of his heart laboring but also hesitant. Was he forgetting something?

Of course he was. Jack was experiencing many of his life's last sensations and emotions. Yet he did not know. He did not pause to savor, to think: this is the taste of warm beer, bitter yet pleasant; this is the holy hush of snow falling; this is the unique sibilance of an empty potato chip bag being crushed into the trash.

Instead, there would be no last words, no consummate gesture, no muttered prayer. Jack did not know that this was his one opportunity to say good-bye.

He glanced into his son's room, but the boy was reading and Jack did not interrupt. He passed his daughter's room, missed her a moment, then went into the bathroom to brush his teeth.

"It's snowing," Jack called through the open door to his wife. "Really coming down."

But when he entered the bedroom Jack saw that she was already asleep. A novel lay open on her lap. He placed the book on the bedside table facedown but still open, so as not to lose her place. It was a little gesture, miniscule really. But she would notice it when she moved the novel again the following night, putting it away on a shelf—she would set aside all reading for many months. At that moment twenty-four hours later, her world having changed utterly, Jack's care over so small a thing would touch her in a deep and previously unknown place. For now, though, she dozed.

Jack climbed into bed and shut off the light. Six hours left. Did his mind, then, turn over the lessons of his life? Did Jack's soul ache at all he was about to lose, so that he reached for his wife and sought the comfort of one last embrace? Did he fear what might come after death—a reckoning perhaps, or bliss, or nothing at all?

No, Jack remembered that the mortgage was due on the third, Wednesday, and he would have to drop off the check on the way to work to avoid paying the late fee.

He shifted his pillow. Lately he'd been folding it over to raise his head while he slept. It helped him breathe, and his wife said he snored less. Jack felt a mild indigestion, that December Monday nearing midnight, but he ignored it and the sensation soon passed.

Then there was only the dark, the quiet house, and in time, dreams. Even on the cusp of ceasing to exist, there are dreams.

THE ALARM BUZZED in darkness and Jack slapped it off: 5:45 A.M. Forty minutes left. Out the window he saw six inches of fresh snow.

Jack was born on April 8. He and his wife celebrated their August 1 anniversary twenty-nine times. He observed holidays and remembered Mother's Days and kids' birthdays and anniversaries of starting jobs. Jack oriented the compass of time with meaningful dates throughout the year. Yet never had he given a moment's thought to his life's fifty-five unremarkable December 2s. Jack's family will remember, though. His son will note the date solemnly every year, honoring his father while in turn ignoring the May 25 that waits with cold patience for him.

Down in the kitchen Jack lit a cigarette, squinting against its smoke as he dug through the hall closet for his boots and parka. A slug of coffee, and out he shuffled into the gray morning. Grabbing a snow shovel, Jack started at the garage and worked his way back. The first few pulls tightened his shoulders. The stuff was heavy. Upstairs the bathroom light went on, meaning his wife was awake, and he began to hurry.

Jack was halfway home when he felt one of his smoking coughs coming on. He straightened, trying to deep-breathe it away. But the air felt as though it went somewhere other than into his lungs, down into his left arm somehow. And when he exhaled, in the place where the breath had been there was a powerful ache. Jack frowned at his arm as if it belonged to someone else. The pain intensified. He leaned the shovel against himself and rubbed his shoulder. How could so small an exertion hurt so much?

A sledgehammer of pain struck Jack in the chest. His body seemed to fold around it. He clutched the shovel for balance, as if staying upright were the most important thing imaginable. Then Jack's knees buckled, slamming his face down on the shovel's handle and giving him an instant nosebleed. He leaned to the right, curling around the massive stab in his core. The snow, with an arc of red from his nose, cushioned his fall.

Whatever was happening, Jack thought, it was going to take over the day. The mortgage payment would definitely be late. Already the world was developing a vagueness. The cold against his cheek, the tightness in his lungs—they grew distant. The early daylight in some kind of ebb. Even the pain became strangely remote.

Jack's eyes roved, and he thought to ask: "Anyone?"

Minutes later his wife, humming along with the radio, glanced out the bathroom window. She saw Jack's form, prone amid a spray of red. She screamed and screamed.

WHAT IS THE IMPRINT a body makes when it falls? Later that morning, when Jack was lifted from where he lay, with all the care that experts in that grim line of work can provide while nearby a stricken wife and son watch, the outline he left was no snow angel. No, if you take a man in a loose parka and tip him sideways with a shovel in his hand, the shape that remains is strange but familiar: a human form, hooded and cloaked, and in his merciless grip the tool that spares no one, the scythe.

CHAPTER TWO

THIS IS THE NEWS

In 1976 that is how most Americans died. Death came suddenly, without warning or reprieve, life's largest pill swallowed all in one gulp.

The nation's leading cause of death for much of the past century has been heart disease, and its most common manifestation in 1976 was the heart attack. Back then Americans suffered more than 750,000 heart attacks annually. Stroke—the bursting of a blood vessel in the brain—was another major cause of death. Accidents rounded out the top tier of the list.

A generation ago life ended swiftly. Death fell upon most people with nearly the speed and severity of a guillotine blade.

It is no longer so. Over the past thirty years the rapid causes of death have declined, while gradual causes have grown exponentially. Most people today do not die suddenly; they die incrementally.

Not only is the manner of death changing, but the change is accelerating. A few numbers describe the transformation succinctly.

- First the big one: Deaths from heart attack now occur at a rate 61 percent below that of thirty years ago.

- Stroke fatalities have plummeted, too, by 71 percent in the past thirty years.

- The rate of fatalities from accidents has plunged 36 percent.

The way we die has been utterly altered.

Today people's dying occurs gradually, from sicknesses that take their lives by degrees. In a recent fifteen-year span, deaths from chronic respiratory disease increased 77 percent. Fatalities from Alzheimer's disease have doubled since 1980. Some 24.3 million people have that illness today, living an average of eight years, and the number is expected to reach 42.3 million in 2020.

The list of gradual killers is long and growing. People now succumb to congestive heart failure, lung disease, diabetes that leads to kidney failure, ALS (or Lou Gehrig's disease), Parkinson's, osteoporosis that results in falls, confusion, and immobility. Today people face a whole battalion of incremental illnesses. AIDS is the brutal newcomer—unheard-of in 1976, the leading killer of twenty-five- to forty-four-year-olds in 1995, and still among the top causes for that age group. But the granddaddy of them all is cancer.

Despite decades of research, yielding near-heroic advances in detection, diagnosis, and treatment, cancer fatalities in the past thirty years have increased 22 percent. Smoking offers a tempting target for blame. Cancers from tobacco take about 180,000 people's lives each year. But cigarettes are only part of the problem. The panoply of various carcinomas, myelomas, and melanomas now accounts for almost 550,000 deaths in America yearly.

The situation will undoubtedly worsen. More than 16 million people were diagnosed with cancer between 1990 and 1997. The American Cancer Society estimates that the odds of Americans having cancer sometime in their life is one in two for men and one in three for women. If current trends continue, by 2010 cancer may replace heart disease as the nation's leading killer.

Fathoming this change from fast to gradual dying takes more than numbers. It requires examining the human experience in both 1976 and now. To begin with, why did Jack and millions of his contemporaries die as they did? Why was death so often sudden?

From a medical standpoint, with today's knowledge of nutrition, the reasons are not mysterious. The human body evolved over eons into an intricate machine whose expected fuel is fruits, vegetables, legumes, nuts, meat, and, since the last Ice Age ended ten thousand years ago, a modicum of wheat, corn, and rice. Food was abundant only seasonally, while migration or at least nomadism was a way of life. In the epochs before domesticated meat sources, those centuries of hunting wild prey with spears and traps, the body's metabolism adapted to store any caloric surplus in the form of fat—which could be broken down during subsequent starving times into fuel again.

That plan remains the evolutionary strategy of all the human bodies now making their way through our entirely different contemporary world. Reduce the greens in that body's intake, add dairy and processed carbohydrates, make meat a daily part of the diet, shovel in sugar and oils, provide a steady supply for the appetite, and on top of all this turn the hunter-gatherer into a mostly sedentary being, and the result is both unfortunate and predictable. The machine stores fat to its own detriment, while the body's strategy for nomadic survival becomes a fatal anachronism. Evolution did not anticipate nine to five. Evolution has no reply to TV.

Thus, the symptoms that conscripted Jack marched a whole population to its grave. In 1976 men dropped from heart attacks not only while shoveling snow but also while mucking the barn, climbing stairs, working the assembly line, playing golf, stacking wood, mowing the lawn, making love.

Women, too, suffered heart attacks by the tens of thousands each year, although typically at a later age and under circumstances reflective of the more domestic life they led a generation ago. In fact, despite all the worthwhile activism about breast cancer, heart disease remains the leading killer of women in America—even though heart attacks are more commonly associated with type-A executives and other men whose bodies are in general disrepair.

Think of poor Jack. After decades of a diet with too much sugar, he may be a borderline diabetic. He smokes, which damages lungs, circulation, the immune system, and more. Junk food has exacerbated a cholesterol problem. What Jack calls sluggishness is really clogged arteries. His habit of folding his pillow is actually an unwitting adaptation to the circulatory problems that accompany early congestive heart disease.

Jack's intelligence is failing him, too. He knows he should live healthier but does not act on that knowledge. He knows he should see a doctor but suspects the result will dictate changes in lifestyle that Jack does not want to make. Rationalizing his behavior is easily done. Most Americans have known someone like Jack.

The pattern was similar for those who fell victim to sudden illnesses not involving the heart. The runner-up cause of death thirty years ago was stroke. All it takes is cholesterol. This pale yellow material builds up in the soft corridors of blood vessels, then calcifies like dried soap, thereby narrowing the passageway. The bottleneck of blood upstream of the clog forces the artery to burst. The brain bleeds into itself. If the hemorrhage is severe, or the artery serves a crucial enough region of the brain, life ends swiftly. If not, the surviving body is weakened by such effects as partial paralysis or an inability to swallow, shortening the remaining life.

Despite the grimness of heart attacks and strokes, sensible people could argue that sudden death had its merits: no bankrupting medical expenses, no caretaking burden for busy adult children, only brief suffering for the victim, no macabre preparation by family and friends.

All true. But this is an incomplete picture. The positives of rapid death came at a high and irrevocable price.

Foremost, for survivors—the family members, neighbors, and coworkers—grief consists of not only loss but also shock. Indeed, the second emotion might overpower the first for months or even years.

This surprise, this unfamiliarity with death across an entire culture, is a relatively new phenomenon. A generation or two earlier, the end of a person's days would not have been so foreign. In the early twentieth century, the majority of Americans still had a connection to rural life. People witnessed death on a regular basis: the beheading of chickens and butchering of pigs, the methodical violence of hunting and trapping, the various accidents and illnesses commonplace on a farm.

Urban culture, too, fostered greater awareness of mortality. Cities used to be divided mainly along ethnic lines, and within those neighborhoods lived people of all ages. Many urban households had multiple generations under one roof, so that from childhood forward, aging and mortality were present and even normal.

In tandem with the twentieth century's economic changes—from booming industrialization to the concentration of wealth to soaring agricultural productivity—a rapid social metamorphosis occurred. Increasingly, Americans lived away from life-and-death rhythms. People left farms by the thousands. Meat came neatly packaged. The erosion of experience with mortality happened in urban settings, too, as city neighborhoods shifted to reflect not ethnicity but socioeconomic status. Today ten nationalities might live on the same block, with the primary common denominator being their income level. Few if any of those households have grandparents and grandchildren under the same roof.

With these changes came a dramatic alteration in attitudes toward ill health and death. Society confined sickness to hospitals. Aged and chronically ill people were placed in "homes" removed from everyday life. Where lives ended reversed, from 75 percent of people dying at home in 1920 to 75 percent dying in hospitals or other institutions in 1994. Death came to be considered either a weakness of character or a failure of medical efforts. Either caskets were closed at wakes or the occupants were made to appear as lifelike as possible—even if that appearance was accomplished by draining the body's interior of blood and painting its exterior with cosmetics.

Thus Jack's wife and son typified their culture when they suffered not only his dying but also the brutal surprise of it. They had no education in the concept of utter finality, nor preparation for seeing anyone's unpainted corpse, much less that of their loved one. When Jack's arm flopped off the stretcher as he was being carried away that morning, it was as lifeless a thing as they had ever seen. The swiftness of his death caused a genuine, enduring hurt that compounded the loss.

Sudden death had spiritual negatives, too. Jack had no chance to prepare to meet his maker, in whatever faith and fashion he deemed right. He had no opportunity to declare what mattered most to him, or ask the questions a dying man yearns to have answered.

For their part, Jack's family members had to reckon with all that was incomplete between them emotionally. His son would never forgive himself for reading a book that night instead of staying up to watch the fourth quarter as his father had asked. Jack's wife would forever lament that she had fallen asleep over her novel. His daughter would feel that if only she had been home, since she was an early riser like her father, she might have called for help sooner.

Sudden death's drawbacks were not only spiritual and emotional, they were financial. Jack's will, written when he and his wife were expecting their first child, was almost uselessly out-of-date. Tax laws had changed. They'd bought a larger house. Whether his pension would pass intact to his wife was in question. Despite Jack's life of hard work, her financial future was uncertain.

Throughout that small family unit, its members bonded with new intensity by their shared grief, the impact of Jack's sudden death would reverberate. "If only we had known," they would lament, as would the loved ones of millions of people just like Jack. "If only there had been some warning."

On one level, no warning is needed. Life is fatal. Death is not a medical event, but a natural one. In a symmetry that would be elegant were it not so sad, it is exactly as commonplace as birth.

But that is a metaphysical reality, not a practical one. After all, we know that earthquakes will strike certain locations someday, but that does not stop us from building cities on fault lines. Whether of ground tremors or heart attacks, an approximate prediction would be a priceless advantage. A warning allows time to anticipate, and perhaps prevent, much of the anguish.

In fact, the period of preparation has arrived. This is the news. This is the opportunity.

AMERICAN SOCIETY HAS SEEN many dramatic changes, good and ill, in the past generation. Feminism's victories have brought women into all strata of the workforce. Wealth is concentrated in the hands of fewer people. The Internet has made information a commodity both worldwide and instantaneous. The traditional family has been replaced by a wide variety of household structures. Racial diversity has grown. Homelessness has spread. Soviet communism fell.

Yet the largest societal change in America in recent years has been the transformation of death. It is larger than these other trends because it touches every person. And its impact is all the more dramatic because, aside from medical journals and books on coping with grief, it has gone unremarked upon and comes as a tragic surprise for millions of Americans every year. Indeed, the seismic shift in dying has altered neither public policy nor individuals' behavior.

The change, for a growing number of people every day, is this: dying today is gradual. For the first time in human history, we can anticipate our mortality. We can watch its slow approach. We can look it in the eye.

Quite apart from the statistics cited earlier, people know that dying is different today simply from their own experience. They mourn the friend who found a lump in her breast and lymph nodes, then underwent chemo, radiation, and surgery, and eighteen months later was dead. They recall the neighbor who began acting erratically, later could not finish a sentence and, after a cruelly long decline with his body sound but his mind absent, died unable to recognize his own family. People know the smoker with congestive heart failure who took years to slip from pale skin and cold fingers to a life tethered to an oxygen tank to dying in his nursing-home bed. They remember the diabetic who ignored symptoms until it was too late, surviving after kidney failure thanks only to the mixed blessing of dialysis every few days and spending years on the transplant list only to die before a matching donor could be found. They know the unfortunate soul whose advanced Parkinson's lasted ten years, or whose Lou Gehrig's disease took away one function and one piece of dignity at a time. They watched a person far too young waste away from AIDS.

Yes, gradual death has its own savagery. Its result is no less final than a sudden passing. But death by degrees does mean that *dying* is different. It takes months, not minutes. For a rapidly growing number of people, dying has become a process.

What that transformation means, its implications for doctors and patients and families, its significance for the people you love and one day for you, are the central concerns of this book. When dying is a process, the manner and meaning of a person's final days are not left wholly to chance. There are options and opportunities; there are choices.

TO UNDERSTAND THE ENORMOUS POTENTIAL that now exists in the dying process, and to learn how to maximize that opportunity, it is instructive first to contemplate how the change in death occurred. The survival of thousands of Jacks is no accident. And to their loved ones, given the priceless gift of additional years, death's change is also no small matter.

Medical advances offer some explanation. Beta-blocker drugs that prevent heart attacks, for example, are post-1976 medicines. Prescription drugs have helped treat incremental illnesses, too, from tamoxifen thwarting breast cancer to AZT's success in slowing the onslaught of HIV. Medical researchers predict gains against all manner of diseases once they grasp a fuller understanding of DNA—a day they herald as fast approaching because the mapping of the human genome finished three years ahead of schedule.

But medical discoveries are only part of the story. A more complete answer is that Americans have sought—nay, demanded—better delivery of the medical capacity that already exists, and better access to it regardless of cost, because they believe this improvement will give them longer and healthier lives.

They are not always right. Replacing an aging ambulance with a medevac helicopter is no substitute for sensible eating and regular exercise. But when it comes to sudden death, the demand for improved delivery of care—an insistence on better service—has made a demonstrable difference. The change has come at many levels of society, from government programs to hospital facilities to communication tools to skills that Americans have learned for themselves, all to thwart sudden death.

Just consider Jack lying on his front walk. If his heart attack takes place in 2006 instead of 1976, his wife will be no less upset when she sees his prostrate form. But now she can grab the phone and dial 911. That emergency communication system did not exist in 1976. Now it is nearly nationwide, reaching into even the country's most rural areas. The dispatcher relays Jack's crisis to a local team of emergency medical technicians. The prevalence of these health workers illustrates how dramatically change has come. The first call for medical personnel specialized in rapid-response trauma care came in an executive order by President Lyndon Johnson. He had learned that the nation's new 43,000-mile interstate highway system was causing accidents that overwhelmed rudimentary ambulances, sheriffs, and highway patrols. In the wake of Johnson's order, the first candidates for the position of emergency medical technician, some 1,500 strong, took their certification test on October 29 and 30, 1971. By late 2003, the United States had 887,523 emergency medical service practitioners. They were rolling in 54,339 ground ambulance crews, backed up by several hundred air medical transport services. This medical cavalry is trained, tested, and equipped and is available on twenty-four-hour call because the communities they serve both demand it and are willing to pay the taxes to make it possible.

After calling, Jack's twenty-first-century family does not wait passively. His son begins the vigorous chest massage and breathing support known as cardiopulmonary resuscitation, or CPR. There are no national registries of people who have learned this rescue technique, so an exact count is not available. But the Red Cross, the American Heart Association, and local health clubs and safety groups have taught CPR to millions of people since 1976. Before a summer lifeguarding job, Jack's son spent a Saturday learning CPR himself. And thus he knows that even if he cannot restart his father's heart, he may force some oxygen into his brain, minimizing the damage should his father regain consciousness.

The rescue squad reaches Jack's house in minutes. One EMT works on Jack while another interviews the family for his medical history. She ushers Jack's wife and son back into the house, sparing them unpleasant images. Later she will contact a counselor to help them cope with the emotions of that day and the fears that may visit afterward.

Meanwhile the first EMT has scissored open Jack's shirt and is preparing to shock his chest with two metal conductive paddles. Many heart attacks are the result of a blockage in one of the blood vessels that supply the heart muscle. The organ's four chambers lose their timing relative to one another. In uncoordinated panic, they writhe. The arrhythmia prevents blood from flowing as it should to deliver oxygen to the brain and other vital organs. An electrical jolt can reorient the heart's quadrants, reestablishing the rhythm that sustains life.

The devices that provide this shock are called defibrillators, and they have been around for decades. In 1976, however, they were available only in hospitals. The equipment was expensive, needed electricity to function, and required a trained technician. They also weighed 110 pounds. Today defibrillators cost a few thousand dollars and run on portable batteries. Roughly the size of a laptop computer, they weigh less than eight pounds. Beyond the ambulances that carry them as a matter of course, defibrillators can be found everywhere from health-club locker rooms to corporate offices to the shuttle bus stops at Disney World. Even home defibrillators have come onto the consumer market.

So the EMT in 2006 gives Jack's chest a burst of electricity. The heart searches for its beat, hesitates, and then regains a rhythm that is feeble but self-sustaining. The technician promptly attaches a dozen electrocardiograph leads to Jack's chest, again using recently portable equipment to obtain information that makes rapid diagnosis possible. He sends the data ahead to the hospital, one more time employing new technology.

Then the EMT signals to his partner, and together they load Jack into the ambulance. Jack's wife follows in her car, her son in the passenger seat, using his own post-1976 device, a cell phone, to call his sister.

At the hospital Jack is admitted. In 1976 the medical community was debating how to treat heart attacks. Today the argument has largely ended. Aspirin's value in preventing further blood-vessel blockages, for example, is uncontested. In fact, when the national hospital accrediting organization wants a snapshot of heart-attack treatment, it measures what percent of patients receive aspirin within twenty-four hours of admission.

If Jack lives near a community hospital, he will receive an anticlotting drug with a better than 90 percent success rate. If Jack lives near a major medical center, he will be rushed to a cardiac catheterization lab. There a physician, guided by an overhead X-ray camera, will puncture Jack's blockage with a tiny wire, then inflate a balloon in the artery to open the flow. The surgeon may also insert tiny wire meshes called stents to prevent future clogs. This approach nearly eliminates the risk of another heart attack. Thus 95 percent of the patients survive.

Think of this achievement. About 6.4 million people now survive angina chest pain *each year,* while an additional 700,000 people survive a heart attack *each year*.

Even though many people do not receive ideal care quickly enough, medical intervention in heart disease saves literally millions of lives. In

2002 alone there were 2,057 heart transplants, 93,000 heart-valve replacements, and 515,000 cardiac-bypass procedures. The success of these procedures is astonishing: Right now there are 13 million victims of heart disease alive in the United States.

Treatment of strokes, the second-leading cause of death in 1976, remains complex. It's not as simple as giving aspirin, and stroke remains a major cause of permanent disability. Still, there have been gains. About 700,000 Americans still suffer a stroke each year. Some 530,000 of them survive. Consequently, about 5.4 million stroke survivors are alive in America today.

The point is that progress in the fight against sudden death is not solely a result of medical advances. It is a result of spending huge sums to battle the causes: The American Heart Association estimates the cost of heart disease and stroke at $393.5 billion annually. Another factor that must not be underestimated, even in light of such a massive expenditure, is the consumer-driven improvement in delivery of existing medical tools.

The decline in accidental deaths follows this pattern. Although recent years have brought many lifesaving improvements in emergency medicine, the factors in reducing accidental fatalities are as varied as bike helmets and flotation vests, occupational-hazard protections in factories, car-safety recalls, and utilities' more vigilant pruning of trees alongside power lines.

The evidence of a national mobilization against sudden death is considerable: At about the same time as Lyndon Johnson's order that led to EMTs, the Red Cross began offering lifeguarding courses to reduce drownings. Starting with the National Traffic and Motor Vehicle Safety Act, Congress began a series of mandated safety standards, from compelling auto manufacturers to include seat belts to requiring children in the 1990s to ride in car seats. The Federal Aviation Administration began investigating air crashes in painstaking reconstructive detail; today no other form of mass transportation is safer. The food supply had to meet higher standards under the Wholesale Meat Act and the Wholesale Poultry Products Act.

In fact, Washington repeatedly bolstered the push for a safer America. Pollution that caused illness or death diminished under the Clean Water Act and the Safe Drinking Water Act. When Congress created the Consumer Products Safety Commission, establishing government standards in areas as varied as medicine bottle caps and children's pajamas, the rate of death and injury from accidents fell 20 percent in a decade.

Courtrooms have been a factor, too. It's easy to argue that American society has become too litigious. Yet one welcome side effect of consumer and employee lawsuits has been improved product and workplace safety.

From 2002 to 2003 alone, the rate of deaths due to injury on the job fell 13 percent.

Quantifying the actual number of lives saved is harder than with heart attacks or strokes. Statisticians can't measure a death that didn't occur. But the impact on American lives can certainly be counted in the tens of thousands each year.

How did accidents decline? People demanded it. And they took personal responsibility, buying safer cars and suing unsafe manufacturers while developing skills for their own benefit. How did heart attacks and strokes decline? The same way, from consumer demand coupled with changed public behavior.

So it is that life expectancy in America continues to grow. Social advocacy, governmental policy, and personal action combine—and succeed. In 1900 the average American lived to be forty-seven. His counterpart in 2000 lived to be seventy-five, a single-century jump of twenty-eight years. Yet the latest data, from late 2005, indicates an even better average expectancy of 77.6 years. Note, too, that the extension of life is accelerating: Almost two-thirds of the gain—nearly two decades of life—has been accomplished since 1960 as a result of the mobilization against sudden death. That is what such a comprehensive societal response can bring: eighteen years.

Some demographers argue that using average life expectancy may actually understate the gains. Another statistic may be more telling: In 2000 there were 4.2 million Americans aged eighty-five or older; by 2030, when the 1950s baby boomers reach old age, the number of people over eighty-five will have more than doubled, to 9 million.

It is a signal accomplishment of the postwar generation that despite the public's many complaints about the cost and complexity of medical care, and despite the well-documented decline in exercise rates and increase in obesity, people today simply live longer.

Consider the 2006 Jack, recovering from his heart attack on that Tuesday afternoon. His wife and son stand at his intensive-care bedside. His daughter is on a plane. Bo, his work buddy, paces in the hall. With the blocked artery now open, Jack actually feels better, stronger, and more alert than when he got out of bed that morning. Six hours after his heart stopped, Jack blinks his eyes open. Manifesting an excess of joy, everyone weeps.

CHAPTER THREE

A BABY AND
A BASKETBALL GAME

J ack's eyes also have been opened to the value of his life. For now he
has cheated death, and his discoveries are instructive.

Foremost, he has received a warning. Jack cannot unlearn what
he has discovered about his habits. He must manage his sugar intake and
reduce fats. He must take drugs for his blood pressure. He must become
physically active, to shed pounds and gain cardiovascular capacity. Somehow he must put the Camels down for good.

Remarkably, Jack does each of these things to some extent. Fear of
death, an acute sense of how near he came, and the fragility he feels life
now possesses persuade him to make healthier choices. Every day after
lunch, instead of smoking a butt, he strolls the sidewalks around his
workplace, returning energized for the afternoon ahead. He can see modest results in his waistline, too. Jack has developed a keen appreciation for
what medicine can do. It can bestow that rarest of jewels, a second
chance.

Awakened to the value of his days, Jack makes the most of them. He
watches his studious son obtain a degree. He walks his daughter down the
aisle. He celebrates anniversaries with his wife. He reaches retirement,
experiencing the aimlessness, adjustment, then liberation of free time.

Not everything is sentimental, though. Jack monitors his weight with
a vigilance approaching ferocity. He updates his will, increases his life insurance, selects a burial plot. As winter nears, he buys a snow blower.

Is there any way to assign a value to these years? Not really. It is all beyond tallying. Living may even be more precious to Jack than it was before his heart attack. Time contains a warmth it did not possess then, because now life's limits are never forgotten.

Eventually Jack's body begins to wane. The factors that triggered the heart attack reassert themselves. Or diabetes weakens his circulation, bringing foot sores that won't heal and thus making him sedentary. Or blood-pressure problems require stronger drugs, with greater side effects. In the most likely scenario, cancer strikes.

Jack approves removal of the offending tissue—part of his colon, say. He undergoes chemotherapy, though the medicinal poison is so intense that he often confuses its effects with the disease. He receives radiation, which leaves him feeling parched to the point of exhaustion. Often he sees dismay on the faces of loved ones when they watch what he is enduring. Jack's opinion of medical intervention is, to put it gently, evolving.

Maybe Jack earns another year or so. But then his kidneys falter. Or his lungs begin to weaken. Or he experiences confusion about where he is. Or the cancer returns. The machine is older, after all. It will not run forever.

Eventually Jack's fate cannot be denied. Maybe his doctor informs him that nothing more can be done. Maybe his wife asks him, before the next round of chemo, to consider how much more he wants to put himself through. Maybe Jack himself recognizes that the specter he cheated all those years ago had always planned to return.

But Jack has faced death before, and he feels equipped to face it again. He opts out of further intervention. He asks his doctor for help with pain, and his friends and family for help with everything else. As Jack's end approaches, they surprise him.

There is the Sunday morning his son stops by, offhandedly mentions an article he saw in the newspaper, and, prompted by Jack's questions, finds the story and reads it to him. So begins a weekly routine, son reading to father, that will last as long as Jack lives.

There is the clergyman who pays a visit to ask after Jack's health, and the conversation lasts hours. Then Jack spends a little time each day contemplating his place in the larger order of things, and preparing his spirit for a transition from the tangible and known to the intangible and unknown.

There is the evening, late in Jack's illness, when his wife enters the room to find his mouth fallen open and parched, and she dips her pinkie in a glass of water and spreads it around his lips and over his tongue. Jack awakens and smiles at her weakly. They know that all of their years together do not approach the level of intimacy they share now.

There is the weekday when Jack is sleeping and his daughter places on his diminished chest a baby, eight pounds of squalling aliveness, a grandson, and Jack finds himself suddenly alert and fully present, holding this incomparable creature who bears his name, John, and feeling all in the same instant the swift passage of years, pride in his daughter, nostalgia for his own children's infancy, and delight at the tiny fingers.

Near the end there is the nurse who bathes him and monitors his pain and wipes his bottom with no hesitancy or constraint. Dimly as Jack perceives her, the nurse's matter-of-factness feels like a new kind of compassion.

Not everyone is so heroic. Many people during that long decline are frightened of Jack. Neighbors, former coworkers, some relatives, they know perfectly well they cannot catch cancer from him. But strong emotions? Those are highly contagious. So some people withdraw, telling themselves they do not want to impose or interfere.

It is all rationalization. They're actually terrified of saying or doing the wrong thing, as if a faux pas could kill someone. They are also afraid because seeing Jack may force them to contemplate, however briefly, their own mortality. It is one of the first losses Jack must accept, the disappearance of acquaintances who believe they are unequipped to reckon with what they actually will all face in due time.

Jack's former coworker Bo, for example, feels a conflict almost daily between wanting to call Jack to see how he's doing and thinking it would be an intrusion. One Saturday Bo bumps into Jack's wife at the grocery store. He asks about his pal, and she insists that he stop by that afternoon. Bo hesitates but agrees. When he arrives at Jack's house Bo rings the doorbell, then shuffles his feet like a teenager taking a cheerleader on their first date.

Jack's wife opens the door, welcomes Bo, and, though she can feel his reluctance, guides him into the living room. Jack is skeletal there on the couch, eyes dimmed and skin waxy. But he raises his arm to shake hands, tells Bo how glad he is to see him, invites him to join him in watching a Celtics game.

Bo sits on the edge of a chair, accepts the offer of a beer. Jack says lately he's lost the taste for beer, and jokes that some fates are worse than death. Bo finds himself chuckling. He tells Jack a few jokes he's heard lately, mostly obscene, and before long the two of them are guffawing.

The Celtics win. Jack teases Bo a bit about his Lakers, and the banter's familiarity is like reassurance. Almost under his breath Jack says he regrets never seeing his team play in person. Then it's time to leave. Bo stands, and the awkwardness returns. But it's different, too, as though some boundary has been crossed.

On the drive home Bo can't stop thinking, and soon he has a plan. On Monday morning Bo calls the Celtics' box office and explains his idea. When it comes to the wishes of a dying man, Bo discovers, special treatment is not hard to arrange.

By the time Bo next visits Jack, the plan is complete. They will rent a van that can accommodate Jack's wheelchair. They will drive to Boston to watch the Celtics play the Bulls. If they arrive early, they can watch some of the team's warm-up. Jack is reluctant, until his wife promises to go, too.

On the big day, the arena staff is eager to ensure a success. They take Jack by elevator down to courtside. Peering up at the stands all around, the retired jerseys hanging in the rafters, Jack tells Bo he cannot believe he is actually there.

Jack is bright-eyed at the tip-off, pivoting in his chair to follow the action. Early in the second half, though, his energy flags. Jack's wife catches Bo's eye, and they decide without a word.

"I'm so sorry," Jack says on the way to the van, his head lolling.

"About what?" Bo replies. "Forget it. That was great."

Back at the hotel Bo hoists Jack on and off the toilet, then lifts him into bed. This is all new territory for him. There's a pause, and the two men regard each other.

"Great day," Jack says.

"Got that right," Bo answers. He reaches to shake hands, but Jack pulls him down into a hug. Bo cannot remember the last time he and another grown man hugged. Strong squeeze for such a frail guy, too.

Later that day, that month, and periodically for the rest of his life, Bo will recall the Boston trip and experience an unusual set of emotions. He almost has to remind himself that Jack's illness was sad, because his strongest feeling is the gratification that comes from helping a dying person to live well. Later Jack's wife will thank Bo, and he will respond that he should be thanking her for the experience.

Toward the end Jack sleeps. Whenever he opens his eyes his wife is present. She is as steady as the sun. If he tries to thank her, she shushes him. They spend more time looking into each other's eyes than they did while courting.

Jack dies in the morning, a Friday, July 19. The passage from life to death is so slight, his family cannot tell for certain when Jack has gone. But then it is evident. There is no crisis, though, no emergency. Only a sober time when his wife and children cry for a while. But they are calm. Jack's work is done. The funeral is already prepared. There are a few calls to be made. But they are calm.

Jack's wife hugs her children in the hallway. She tells them how lucky she feels.

CHAPTER FOUR

A DOG IS BETTER
THAN A PILL

Actually, Jack is the lucky one. His death was virtually ideal. It contained pain, certainly, and ended in loss. But it also possessed unique pleasures, thanks to the opportunity Jack and his family had to make meaningful choices. His process exemplifies what is possible, how the close of a life can be personalized, how shaping the journey to the traveler can provide solace to the dying and comfort to those who remain.

Yet deaths like Jack's are rare. Despite people's intentions, they do not die as Jack did. Here are the realities of where and how Americans die.

Depending on the region of the country, between 50 and 60 percent of people's lives end in hospitals. They go to these institutions for advanced care like surgery or because of an emergency or for medical equipment such as ventilators and feeding tubes. If they are near death, these patients typically land in intensive care. However, many terminally ill patients come to wish that their desire for late-stage heroic interventions had gone ungranted.

There is nothing wrong with hospitals, of course, nor with people who work in ICUs. On the contrary, intensive care saves thousands of lives each year. Countless trauma patients would not recover without the powerful tools and specialized expertise of intensive care.

Yet there may be a great deal wrong with using intensive medicine on a person whose death is certain and near. To begin with, for the patient, everyone in the ICU is a stranger. For the family, the head clinician comes into the patient's room, introduces himself, and promises to have the unit's other doctors stop by during their shift. Those visits may actually happen over the next few days, if the unit is not too crowded. Even if family members can keep these people straight, though, not one of the doctors knows the slightest nonmedical thing about the patient. There is negligible opportunity to personalize the care, much less help the sick person pass time in a fulfilling way. Visitation hours are limited, and there is little flexibility for making the room more comfortable or comforting. If the patient is conscious as he dies, breath by dwindling breath, he is also monumentally bored.

It is not crass to consider as well the cost of dying this way. An ICU bed costs about two thousand dollars a day, not counting lab tests and special equipment fees. That burden falls in part on health insurers (and thus whoever pays the premiums) and in part on taxpayers (when Medicare pays ICU bills). But the financial strain is heaviest on patients' loved ones. Medical bills—not credit cards—are the leading cause of bankruptcy in America. A 1995 study found that 31 percent of the families of dying people spent "all or most of their savings" on the patients' hospital care.

This extravagance would be worthwhile if it resulted in a better experience for the person who is dying. But definitive research has found the opposite to be the case. Half of American patients who died in hospitals, one authoritative study found, experienced "moderate or severe pain at least half the time" during their final days.

Those last hours were not filled with quiet dignity and compassion, either. The same study found that 38 percent of patients who died in hospitals spent ten or more days in intensive care or on a ventilator. Researchers have revealed how unwelcome that level of intervention was to patients and families: 44.9 percent of ICU deaths came after life support was withdrawn or withheld. In essence, people in that situation were almost eager to die.

Sometimes patients try to take control of the situation. They draw up legal documents that either permit another person to speak for them when they cannot or dictate what treatments they want and which they consider excessive.

However, only a fraction of people have these instructions in place. Moreover, ICUs routinely act contrary to these directives, because staffers either are unaware that the documents exist or are too busy to read them. One study found that 70 percent of physicians failed to determine whether dying patients wanted to be resuscitated in an emergency.

The situation is no better in the second most common location where death occurs, nursing homes. About eighteen thousand of them are spread across America, housing almost 2 million people. Today more than 20 percent of Americans' lives end in these facilities, a number almost certain to rise.

There's nothing inherently wrong with nursing homes. They allow for a modicum of personal care, and families generally can visit wherever they wish. But the national nursing shortage, plus cost constraints that lead to fewer staffers being medically trained, has compromised the quality of nursing-home care.

That is not conjecture. The federal agencies that fund and oversee nursing homes make quality information public about individual facilities. Researchers at the University of California in San Francisco collated all that data to provide a national overview. The truth is ugly.

- Residents were strapped down: 11.2 percent of nursing homes used physical restraints "for purposes of discipline or convenience" not related to the patient's medical symptoms.

- Residents were hungry: 9.3 percent of homes provided inadequate food, 7.7 had food that was nutritionally inadequate, 5.3 percent served "infrequent meals," and a stunning 36.2 percent failed to prepare and serve food in a manner sufficiently sanitary to prevent illness.

- Residents were dirty: 19.9 percent of nursing homes had poor housekeeping, while 13.8 percent failed to help people with daily living tasks such as grooming and oral hygiene.

- Residents grew sicker for avoidable reasons: 17.5 percent of nursing homes failed to "ensure that residents without pressure sores did not develop them." Another 11.8 percent failed to treat people with bladder incontinence well enough to prevent lost function and restore what had been lost. Some 18.4 percent of the homes failed to provide a comprehensive plan for residents' care, and 9.3 percent were cited for improper infection control. The general quality of care was deficient in 30.5 percent of the facilities.

- Residents were at risk: 22.4 percent of nursing homes provided insufficient measures to prevent accidents, and 25.5 percent had environmental hazards. Another 24.6 percent had poor professional standards for staff, 13.6 percent hired "unemployable individuals," and 8.6 percent failed to follow proper pharmacy procedures.

- Residents were humiliated: 17.5 percent of nursing homes failed to maintain the dignity of their residents. Another 10.7 percent were deficient in protecting residents' privacy and confidentiality.

Strapped down, hungry, dirty, humiliated—that is the experience of American elders. Each of these scores, not incidentally, reflected a decline in care quality since 1997. The number of problems per facility leapt 40 percent in six years. Living in a high-end home provided no guarantees, either. The number of facilities with no deficiencies at all was 9.5 percent in 2003, less than half the number in 1997.

Regardless of whether consumers know these grim details, they have strong opinions about nursing homes anyway. In a 2001 survey of 3,262 seriously ill patients, only 7 percent said they were "very willing" to live in a nursing home. In fact, 26 percent said they were "very unwilling" to do so. A striking 30 percent said they would "rather die" than live in a nursing home.

Here's the really bad news: According to geriatric-care specialists, 56 percent of Americans alive today will wind up in a nursing home at some point. Of those who stay longer than two weeks, 76 percent will die in that facility. Twenty percent will spend more than five years in a nursing home.

People would rather die than face a fate that, in growing likelihood, certainly awaits them.

Concerned about the downward trend in quality of care during an upward trend in people's reliance on nursing homes, Congressman Henry Waxman of California called for a congressional investigation of the industry. The report was chilling. Over the span of one year almost one-third of nursing homes—5,283 of them, to be exact—were cited for abuse of their residents. The report found that the number of nursing homes cited for abuse was increasing every year. Abuse was verbal, physical, and sexual. Perpetrators sometimes were nursing-home employees and sometimes other residents.

"It would have been intolerable if we had found a hundred cases of abuse," Waxman said. "It is unconscionable that we have found thousands upon thousands."

The tragedy is so commonplace, it has created a market. Now there are companies that offer security cameras for nursing homes. The sales pitch is that families who install surveillance equipment in their loved one's room are really buying protection; abuse is far less likely if it might be captured on video. Lost privacy is considered acceptable if it reduces the odds of harm. This is what elder care has come to. This is what awaits millions of today's healthy Americans.

Between hospitals and nursing homes, the situation has become so dire that in 2003 the National Association of Attorneys General, an organization of the fifty states' top law-enforcement officials, declared end-of-life patient care the top consumer-protection issue in the country.

BECAUSE NEITHER THE PUBLIC NOR policy makers have known that dying has become gradual, they continue to treat the final stages of slow dying mistakenly, as if it were a sudden trauma. Consider two trends. First, the number of hospitals across the country fell from 5,803 in 1980 to 4,895 in 2003, a drop of 16 percent. Second, during that same period the number of intensive-care beds jumped from 54,633 to 60,826—a leap of 11 percent. That happened while Americans were living longer and while more of them were succumbing to incremental illnesses. In other words, the manner of dying and the manner of its treatment have been moving in opposite directions.

So, today there are machines to breathe for the patient, medicines to sustain blood pressure, tubes to provide nutrition, equipment to perform the tasks of the heart, lungs, kidneys, and bladder. Of course, using these devices is imperative if a patient might recover. The question is their usefulness for a person who will never be cured. The technology is so complete, neither a beating heart nor a functioning brain is required to enable a body to persist on this side of what was once considered death. The machines can even keep a body's parts viable after the person has certifiably died; hospitals routinely do this while arranging organ transplants.

When high-tech medicine is most successful in preventing an all-but-certain death, however, it is also most dehumanizing—in the cases when medicine saved a life but not the person. There are now roughly 35,000 people in the United States living in a persistent vegetative state. That's 35,000 people with no consciousness and no chance of recovery, the body's organs kept alive by ventilators and feeding tubes. Imagine the agony for their families. Imagine the expense. And to what gain?

Perhaps these 35,000 lives may yet serve a societal purpose, if their plight awakens people to the change in dying from sudden to gradual and compels society to act upon that knowledge. Aware that death is likely to come slowly, patients could prepare for their passing with deliberation and calm. Families could offer and receive care while helping their loved ones close out their life with peace and unrivaled richness. Friends could provide the best that friendship is, the shared experience and common values. Medical professionals could deliver the kind of care that first led them to choose that line of work, the empathy and intimacy, the respectful treatment of a patient's ultimate trust.

But that is not how it happens. That is not what America has done with gradual death. The profound opportunity is nearly always missed.

Until recent years the only people who knew for certain that death was approaching were criminals facing execution. Indeed, anticipating his life's end, at a fixed time and place and by a predetermined means, was a key component of the condemned man's punishment.

America's attitude toward gradual dying remains locked in that thinking. People unfamiliar with death in any form are unequipped to capitalize on the unique potential of its present manifestation. The result? At a minimum, dying people experience preventable suffering. At the maximum, patients, families, and caregivers miss some of the most precious, compassionate moments life has to offer. We turn to medical technology that invades instead of curing, prolongs instead of healing, at a time when we, across the whole of society, could all be expanding our hearts.

CONSIDERING THIS OPPORTUNITY, some of the obstacles are painfully practical. One example is physicians' worries over getting sued. Doctors routinely perform extra and perhaps unneeded medical actions out of fear that they could face a malpractice suit if they fail to use every treatment option. They likewise do not use the full power of pain medications, out of concern that they could trigger a criminal investigation of their prescribing practices.

Doctors' caution is entirely understandable. Yet surveys confirm that more than 90 percent of Americans want limits on their medical care at the end of life, no long-term feeding tubes or ventilator, for example, if they are never going to regain consciousness. Even more people want their pain managed aggressively. Thus, at the end of life, doctors and patients have directly conflicting purposes.

A further contributor to the problem may be misuse of medical powers. The word *misuse* ordinarily implies questionable motives, but in this instance it means a lack of awareness of how death has changed, and thus a mismatch between what patients need and what they receive.

Health care is typically delivered using one of three clinical models: critical care, for people with traumatic injuries such as those from a car crash; acute care, for people in a physical crisis such as a heart attack; and chronic care, for people who have an ongoing illness that is not in crisis but requires sustained treatment and attention.

In 1976 people struck by the major causes of death needed acute and critical care. They required aggressive interventions and techniques, responding to a sudden crisis and its immediate aftermath. That kind of treatment is precisely what an ICU is expert at delivering. And that expertise has been heroically successful. Today, though, when death is gradual, patients need a chronic-care model. They need more nonclinical services, greater consideration of their emotions, families, and finances. The ICU is as wrong a fit as using sports-medicine techniques to deliver a baby.

"Patients," a Rand Institute study maintains, "must navigate a fragmented care system, offering them a patchwork of uncoordinated services that do not meet their needs. Indeed, the experience of an increasing number of families confirms the point that health care arrangements for persons with chronic illness often do not function smoothly, reliably or well."

Christine Cassel, M.D., writing in the Institute of Medicine's seminal study *Approaching Death,* puts the situation in humble terms: "Increasing understanding of genetics, human biology and longevity should not lead to dreams of near immortality, but rather give us greater respect for the cycle of human life. . . . When medicine can no longer promise an extension of life, people should not fear that their dying will be marked by neglect, care inconsistent with their wishes, or preventable pain and other distress."

The American Medical Association, in a 1996 report, delivered a more unvarnished opinion: "We are concerned about providing overly aggressive, unwarranted care, while care that is optimally suited to the dying person's needs is often not available or is not covered by insurance."

The medical system is not alone in being perplexed by slow dying. Families whose loved ones land in intensive care also find themselves grappling with ethical quandaries that did not exist a generation ago: How much care is enough? When a cure is impossible, does using advanced technology make sense? Who decides when to unplug, and whether doing so is right or wrong? At what point is dropping resistance to death's approach a case of abandonment, and when is it an act of compassion?

The first case to raise these questions in the national consciousness also illustrates how thorny the dilemmas are. Karen Ann Quinlan of New Jersey had a night out with friends shortly after banging her head in a fall. The evidence that she mixed alcohol and drugs, as is commonly believed, is actually equivocal. Whatever the cause, Karen wound up brain-dead. Her family wanted to remove her from the ventilator sustaining her life; her doctors resisted. The case went to the New Jersey Supreme Court, which said the family could disconnect. But Karen's doctors obeyed the court's ruling slowly, weaning her over months so that she could survive.

Karen lived nine more years.

The court ruled in 1976. It is a sign of America's slow recognition of how the manner of dying has changed that similar cases continue to trouble the nation's courts and legislatures. Nearly all evidence indicates that society's response to gradual dying is like a patient whose breathing tube has been inadvertently removed: it is flailing.

- In 1990 right-to-life advocates stormed a Missouri hospital to protest the removal of Nancy Cruzan's feeding tube. Her case was the first end-of-life issue to come before the U.S. Supreme Court, which ruled in favor of tube removal.

- In mid-2003 the Florida legislature introduced and passed in a single day a bill allowing the governor to keep Terry Schiavo—after thirteen years in a vegetative state—attached to a feeding tube her husband said she did not want. Sympathizing with her parents' efforts to keep the tube attached, Congress also passed in one day a bill intended to extend her life. That dispute touched five different courts, including six requests of the U.S. Supreme Court to take the case. (The court consistently declined.) She died within days of her tube removal.

- In Maine, Hawaii, and Vermont voters and legislators narrowly defeated proposals to legalize physician-assisted suicide.

In Oregon such a referendum passed, twice, despite strenuous objections by the American Medical Association. It is now legal in Oregon for a doctor to write a person a prescription that, if taken as directed, will end the patient's life. In the law's first seven years, 326 people received the lethal prescriptions; 208 of them took the drugs and died.

Politicians, physicians, and theologians have hotly debated the implications of physician-assisted suicide. Some say it represents the ultimate in patient empowerment. Others call it a perversion of the tools and goals of medicine. But the mere existence of an initiative to hasten life's end is itself a powerful verdict on the quality of America's treatment of the dying. When people in Oregon, upon considering the end-of-life care available to them, decide they would instead prefer to die, what greater condemnation could there be?

THERE IS ANOTHER WAY. Poll after poll has found that Americans do not want to die in hospitals or nursing homes. Consistently more than 90 percent say they want to die at home, among friends and family, with their pain treated aggressively.

There are organizations in every state that provide exactly this kind of care, through the hospice movement. The guiding premise of hospice is that people's needs at the end of their lives are much more than medical. They are spiritual, financial, emotional, psychological. Hospice strives to deliver the dying experience people say they want, attending to details many patients don't consider until someone asks: Which friends will you allow to visit, and whom do you want kept away? What foods do you want to eat until your appetite wanes? What faith, if any, do you wish to celebrate or observe? What old conflicts do you want to reconcile, and which would you rather leave unresolved? How do you want to balance receiving pain medication with remaining alert for visitors? In the final hours, what music do you want playing at your bedside?

Many people mistakenly believe that hospice is a kind of facility, akin to a nursing home. Hospice is actually a set of beliefs, a philosophy of health care that relies on medical facilities only some of the time.

The first hospice did resemble a nursing home, though it was considerably nicer. Founded by Cicely Saunders on the outskirts of London, St. Christopher's Hospice boasts gardens, a room for taking tea, a chapel. As a nursing student during World War II, Saunders received a thorough instruction in suffering. After the war she obtained a degree in social work, then went to medical school and became an M.D. She opened St. Christopher's in 1967.

The hospice philosophy places the patient at the center of care. That means managing pain is paramount, because pain-free people are far better able to attend to other important business. Medical concerns are only a subset of treatment and do not automatically take precedence over a patient's emotional or spiritual needs. As a result, a team of people is involved in the patient's care—doctors, nurses, social workers, clergy, and often volunteers who meet essential nonmedical needs such as driving people to appointments. The philosophy is not geared solely toward the patient, either. Hospice also attends to the sick person's family, their fears and challenges and grief.

The principles of hospice may seem like common sense, but they actually represent a radical departure from conventional medicine. Ordinary health care is organized around certain settings—the doctor's office, the lab, the hospital. Hospice care is designed in accordance with the patient's wishes, which may be to receive care in one of those places or in a nursing home or, most often, at home. Ordinary health care is about treating disease. Hospice is about caring for individuals. Everyday medicine treats only the person who is afflicted. Hospice treats family members as part of the plan of care.

Unfortunately, too often conventional health care believes that when there is no possibility of recovery, nothing more can be done. People in these systems often find themselves abandoned just when they most need attention and care. Hospice believes that as long as a person continues to live, a great deal can be done. The patient is only as alone as he chooses to be.

Finally, regular health care places people within systems, with schedules for medication and tests, fixed hours for meals, and no time or personnel to provide individualized care. Hospice is all about spoiling the patient, personalizing care down to details as specific as the art on the walls, the content and timing of meals, the music in the air. This approach can turn slow dying into something incredibly loving, calm, and even funny.

Hospice may provide cancer patients, for example, with a wide array of services. They may receive pain-control drugs. They may receive radiation to ease their suffering without aiming for a cure. They may obtain counseling or help from clergy. They may formalize in writing what steps they want taken to prolong their lives in its final days, and which measures they do not want. They may get help managing their household. Their families may receive respite care, as an aide or volunteer visits the home so loved ones can have a few hours' reprieve from caregiving—to shop for groceries, attend to other responsibilities, or just take a break.

When a person's condition worsens, hospice does not embark on futile adventures to prolong the suffering or delay the inevitable. Instead, the focus remains on keeping the patient as comfortable as possible and supporting her family as much as possible. If there is no one available to provide care at home, or family members are too old or ill or otherwise unable to do the job themselves, hospice becomes an inpatient service, a kind of hospital that specializes in caring for people who are dying. Regardless of where they receive services—and here is perhaps the most dramatic break from conventional health care—when people in hospice care enter their lives' final stages, they are not abandoned. They continue to receive care up to and beyond their last breath. When a patient dies, his or her body is treated with respect. The family receives bereavement services if they wish. The people who cared for the patient, too, are given time and means to mourn.

While defining what hospice is, it is important to make two points about what hospice isn't.

First, hospice isn't alternative medicine or an alternative to medicine. Hospice care is directed by a physician and provided primarily by nurses who specialize in end-of-life care. It employs traditional medical tools for treating pain and other symptoms. Hospice is virtually as much its own form of medicine as cardiology or pediatrics.

Moreover, hospice respects the gains against illness that medical advances have wrought. One seasoned hospice leader notes that of the top twenty childhood diseases she encountered while providing terminal care to children in the 1970s, sixteen have since been eradicated. Medical science is a mainstay of hospice care.

Second, hospice is not about surrender or passivity or hurrying death along. Rather it is a vigorous, active effort to make the quality of a person's life as optimal as possible for as long as possible. The hospice ethos is that death occurs in an instant, and until that instant the patient is fully alive and fully deserving of respectful care. Often the quest may involve matters that are completely nonmedical. For example, a person with advanced terminal illness may wish for reconciliation with an estranged loved one. This issue may be paramount in the patient's mind. Regular health care shows little if any interest in such concerns. Hospice care, by contrast, would involve social workers, intermediaries, whatever means the patient approved, in the effort to achieve a reconciliation.

Perhaps the best way to understand hospice, though, is to see it at work.

Florence Wald, the dean of Yale University's School of Nursing, visited Saunders and St. Christopher's in the late 1960s, then founded America's first hospice in 1974. The Connecticut Hospice operated for years in what is now a convent, then moved to a new facility on a rocky point along the shore north of New Haven.

The building looks like an upscale nursing home. Bright rooms have large windows facing the sea. Outdoor promenades offer views of a small harbor, a few piers, the open water of Long Island Sound. There are benches and statues and gulls.

But again, hospice is not about a building. The Connecticut Hospice serves 4,000 people each year in their homes across the state. Patient referrals come from more than one-quarter of Connecticut's 5,600 doctors. The fifty-two-bed building is there to provide care for people who are alone or whose loved ones, for whatever reason—physical, emotional, financial—are unable even with hospice's help to maintain the patient sufficiently well at home. A small woman who cannot turn her obese husband in bed, a man whose eyesight is too poor to make certain he is giving his wife the correct medications, a loved one whose work demands make it impossible to be on hand as much as needed, a widow whose children live on the opposite coast—these are the people who turn to the hospice inpatient facility.

The first sign that the Connecticut Hospice is not an ordinary hospital is Ipsy-Pipsy, a small gray poodle who greets visitors at the front door. He is a therapy dog and has the run of the building. The floors are carpeted. There is no noise of physicians being paged. No medical equipment is visible outside of patient rooms. There is no hospital smell.

The residents live one or two or four to a room. They eat when they are hungry. There are four small libraries and eight fireplaces. Residents gather in common rooms around a piano or a TV, or simply sit with visitors and look at the Atlantic. The largest meeting room, its doorways wide enough to accommodate a hospital bed, does double duty as a place to hold religious services.

When a patient arrives, he, his bed, and IV bags and other equipment are not brought in through a back entrance or secreted in some side corridor. He enters by the front door, in full view. Sometimes the patient looks grim, right on the verge of death.

"You'd be surprised, though," says Rosemary Johnson-Hurzeler, M.P.H., R.N., president and chief executive of the Connecticut Hospice. "Often within a day or two they look remarkably improved, once they start receiving proper pain management and good care."

Some days a guitar player goes to residents' rooms, and it is not unusual to hear singing from down the hall. Music is part of an overall arts program that ranges from crafts therapy to entertainment. In midafternoon a harp player sets up in the hallway, playing quiet Celtic music.

One way the hospice can afford such trimmings is a human resource that undergirds all its work: volunteers. Federal law on Medicare funding for hospice programs requires the involvement of volunteers, as evidence of community support of the mission. The Connecticut Hospice has six hundred volunteers who are deeply involved in patients' nonmedical care, said volunteer director Pat Nowak-Corradino. Their labor in 2003 was valued at $1.8 million.

Many volunteers come forward after the death of a loved one, having witnessed the hospice philosophy at work. But that does not mean they are free of mixed emotions; plenty are intimidated by the idea of being around people who are dying.

"Everybody gets scared," Pat says. Their fears usually are alleviated during the eight-week training program. Besides, "there's always someone here to talk with. And the families always help, by showing their thanks."

Volunteers' fears soon abate as they discover that patient and family needs are neither grim nor taxing. Many tasks are downright practical.

"Today I just gave some people a ride," says Lou Matteo, seventy-three, a volunteer for twenty years. "I brought a wife and sister to visit a man here. It's a little thing, but I get a lot of satisfaction from it, and they're very appreciative."

When a person has a limited time to live, an afternoon spent with appreciative visitors is a jewel. That illustrates how no detail is too minor. For Lou, a retired barber, often his volunteer work involves scissors.

"You would not believe how grateful people can be sometimes," he says. "They're maybe lying in bed, or at least not able to get out. And they couldn't wait to get a haircut." He shakes his head. "They call me a saint or an angel. For a haircut."

Reverend Charles Woody is the facility's resident chaplain. Johnson-Hurzeler, introducing Reverend Woody to a visitor in a corridor, prompts him to "explain what hospice is about."

The chaplain, a large black man with thick glasses, grins, steps back, and begins to sing. The song is about a man who perseveres in life's trials because he knows God trusts him. His faith in God may falter, but God's faith in him remains constant, and that is what sees him through hard times.

Reverend Woody has a strong voice, and he is in no hurry. The hallway harpist stops playing, the noise from nearby rooms ceases, and the chaplain sings three full verses.

When the song ends, Johnson-Hurzeler claps, as does the harpist, and people in rooms up and down the hall. Reverend Woody bows and heads on to his next appointment, still smiling.

On another floor, hospice worker Sister Eleanor Profuto greets visitors by taking their hand in both of her own and drawing them closer. What Reverend Woody's singing implied, she articulates directly.

"I would hope that we invite peace into people's hearts," Sister Eleanor says. "Their vulnerability is so strong. We try to provide a caring presence so that they can consider the four questions: Is there anyone you would like to say thank you to? Is there anyone you want to say 'I love you' to? Is there anyone you want to say 'I'm sorry' to? Is there anyone you want to say 'I forgive you' to?"

She smiles. "Forgiveness is so powerful for these people. It puts wings on the heart."

Some patients, by the time they've determined their answers to the four questions, have become too sick to communicate as they'd like. "So I sit at the bedside and they tell me what to write," Sister Eleanor says. "It's very beautiful, I got to do it this morning, in fact. And sometimes, when people are just ready to enter the new journey, they give me a blessing. It is so powerful, to receive a blessing from them."

Hospice's values reach outside the building, into the community. For example, Artists Who Care, a local philanthropic group, arrived on a recent day with more than a dozen rectangular packages wrapped like presents.

"We knew that in some of the rooms, because patients are away from the windowsill, they don't have a place to put their photographs," explains Dr. Stephanie Wainwright, who does not work at the hospice but participates in Artists Who Care. "We have a wish list on our Web site, so we heard about that problem."

The packages, one for each resident room that has beds away from the windowsill, are homemade bulletin boards.

Such niceties could be misleading, though. Hospice work is not always quiet or predictable. Nor is it all holding hands and singing.

"This is not a nine-to-five sport," Johnson-Hurzeler says. Local doctors with terminal patients use hospice as an on-call resource. Nurses "get called at two in the morning, because we're there at two in the morning."

Meanwhile, providing nonmedical services is not in any way inconsequential, Johnson-Hurzeler says. "If you're throwing up like mad and have your fourth round of chemo the next day, and that one just might make the difference, you need help. You need moral support, sure, but you also need transportation to and from that appointment."

Even with the focus on nonclinical needs, the limitations of the traditional medical culture are a constant concern, says chief medical officer Todd Cote, M.D.

"It's not the angle you would think, of hospitals are bad, doctors are bad," he says. "I don't see that. But people are frustrated; they fear death themselves. Most of all, they don't know what to do or what we do. Just last Saturday a hospital delivered somebody here dead on arrival."

Another hospital contacted Cote for help in withdrawing a patient from a ventilator. It was a community hospital, unaccustomed to a task that nearly always is followed by the patient's death.

"It was a complex case, and they wanted us to help with the weaning. Tomorrow, nine A.M., boom."

Cote folds his arms, shakes his head vehemently. "We said no way. Has anyone dealt with the family's and the caregivers' anticipatory grief? Has anyone talked to the receptionist there, to see how she feels? Preparedness for something like that is profound."

The other kind of hard work that hospice providers know well is raising money.

"We are the oldest hospice in the country, we serve four thousand people a year, we have three hundred and sixty-four people in our care right now, today," Johnson-Hurzeler says. "Yet we have to raise ten percent of our cash from philanthropy. This year that means raising $2.5 million. Our patients are ninety-five percent sicker than all the other hospitals in the country, and we rely on thousands of contributions a year just to stay in business."

The way to win funding and gain converts in a skeptical and territorial medical community, Johnson-Hurzeler says, is with data. It's not easy; normal hospital mortality and morbidity measurements don't apply when 100 percent of hospice's cases end in death. Developing ways of assessing the quality of care, in objective terms, is an ongoing imperative. "Any case we make for the value of hospice must be evidence-based," she says.

Then she gives examples that show how hospice's sights are aimed at both medicinal care and beyond—for instance, in providing a pain-free final chapter to children with terminal illnesses: "Eighty percent of all parents whose firstborn dies wind up divorcing. You can easily imagine why. Not among our pediatrics, though, not here. We have success stories."

Although pediatric deaths can be the most wrenching cases, every family suffers when a loved one is seriously ill. The strain on families can take many forms, Cote says, and when it comes to hospice one common form is fear.

"They're afraid that this is the place to go to die," he says. "But it can be a huge benefit if they've spent a lot of energy taking care of somebody. Now they don't have to worry about day to day, hour to hour. It's all taken care of for them."

Beyond families' relief, though, the greatest gains are for the patients.

"Micky, that's my mini-collie, she's coming to visit," says Linda Werbesky of Meriden, a town about thirty miles away. "A dog is better than a pill." She laughs.

Linda has lived with lung cancer for five years. It has spread to her brain, adrenal gland, and liver. Her wheelchair sits parked in a common room, her family gathered around the table. A tube snakes out of a fold in Linda's robe, draining maroon fluid into a bag on her chair.

"Today I did some craft things. I get lots of company. This place is great."

Linda does not feel that way about her care elsewhere. "I don't want to mention the name of the hospital, but one time they took me for a test, and at the time I was ordered on clear foods only, and I got left in a hallway. I just wanted some Jell-O, I asked for some. People went by, said, 'Oh sure, sure.' Do you know it took five hours? Five hours to get Jell-O? And by the time I got it, it was suppertime."

"It is the simple things that can make all the difference," Dr. Cote interjects. "The Jell-O. Turning a patient in bed. It's not always the fancy medical stuff."

"One of the aides here," Linda continues, "she was done with all of her work the other day, and what does she do? She goes up and down and asks people if they want their nails done."

Linda displays her shaped and polished nails, then drops her voice to a whisper. "In my room there's two people who are dying. They're really going to be gone soon. But even if the family is not there, they treat them so good. That's a real good plus. I've worked in convalescent homes, and they'd snap at patients. Here, no way. The exact opposite. I find that very important."

Good care means both personal services and high-quality medicine.

"Hospice is not about being nice," Johnson-Hurzeler says. "It is about systems shutting down, a body coming apart, and a person needing sophisticated symptom control."

Linda Werbesky is a prime example, Johnson-Hurzeler says. "She was able to talk about Jell-O because she was getting sophisticated pain management so she could be out of bed and alert."

Ethel Fulton arrived at the Connecticut Hospice with what doctors estimated was one week to live. "I have cancer all over my body," the eighty-three-year-old Hamden resident says six weeks later. "When I came here I had so much pain. Within a week they had it under control."

Ethel sits in a recliner by the window, watching waves shatter on the rocks below. "I've been to five different convalescent homes, and there is no comparison with here. I'd rather go out on the street than go back to one of them."

Her immediate concern is a throat infection that makes swallowing difficult. "I have to have my food pureed. But every one of the nurses is here for you."

Ethel has endured a long ordeal, thirteen years from her mastectomy to this chair by the window. The cancer has been slow but unrelenting. "Now it's everywhere, in all my bones, in my spine."

Yet she says she is not anxious about the future. "I haven't asked my doctor how long I have to live. But I know one thing. This is the way to go."

THE CONNECTICUT HOSPICE accomplished some specific things for Ethel Fulton and Linda Werbesky; nationally, the hospice philosophy meets those same goals for thousands of people.

Consider pain. Of hospice patients with cancer, the portion "who suffer unmanageable pain" is 2 percent—versus 50 percent suffering physical pain in hospitals.

Consider location. Seventy-seven percent of hospice patients die at home. Many of the remainder end their lives at residential hospice centers, so the actual tally of hospice patients dying in hospitals and nursing homes is likely under 20 percent.

Consider cost. Hospice reimbursement runs about $120 per day. A bed in the ICU starts at $2,000 a day.

No wonder a National Hospice Organization survey found that 99 percent of hospice patients' families are satisfied with the care.

One potent symbol of hospice's value comes from the Quinlan family. Karen's parents wrote a book about her story, using some of the proceeds to found a hospice in their New Jersey community. Nearly twenty years after his daughter's saga began, Karen's father became a patient in that hospice. He had terminal bone cancer. With a living will to guide his treatment, Joe Quinlan died in the care of the Karen Ann Quinlan Hospice.

In all, it sounds like a solution. Families whose loved ones have received hospice care are nearly evangelical about its capacity to deliver a beautiful death. Indeed, that explains hospice's popularity where the movement began, in Great Britain.

In America, however, hospice is barely a sapling. Fewer than 20 percent of dying people use hospice resources to control and personalize their care. With the potential demand for dignified end-of-life care that exists today, just imagine the flood that will come in 2011 when the first baby boomers reach sixty-five years of age and are able to use hospice resources.

The trends are not encouraging. The number of sites providing hospice care has been increasing at about 3.5 percent a year, and the number of hospice patients has also grown. But the number of intensive care beds also increased, the revenues they generate expanding at a rate averaging $17 billion a year. That means a larger share of the nation's health-care dollars winds up in high-cost, low-quality end-of-life care.

Hospice usage rates vary widely around the country. Rural areas score low, either because there are too few nurse providers or because the widely dispersed financial resources cannot meet the funding needs. Large cities fare poorly, too, perhaps because their academic medical centers accept hospice's role only with reluctance. In New York City in 2002, for example, 12.8 percent of terminally ill patients were found suitable for hospice; one hospice director in the city said it should be closer to 60 percent.

Many people who do enroll in hospice receive only a fraction of its potential benefit. The portion of hospice patients who died within one week of admission has increased 67 percent since 1992. Even hospice's strongest advocates admit that one week is far too brief a time to get pain under control, learn the patient's particular needs, and establish support systems for the family.

These trends raise a central question about living well while dying slowly: If hospice is so effective, so compassionate, and so relatively inexpensive, why don't more people receive this treatment? Since the hospice model aligns so closely with how Americans say they want to be cared for at the end of their lives, why do so few people benefit from it? After all, everyone who goes to the emergency room with a broken leg receives an X-ray. Is end-of-life care so different?

Yes, it is. End-of-life care is different to medical educators, who spend more time teaching students how to deliver a baby than how to deliver an adult into eternity. It is different to health insurers, especially government programs, which will pay for extravagant medical interventions but not the tender loving care people want and deserve in their last days. It is different to hospital administrators, who generate huge revenues from inpatient intensive care units but don't make a nickel if a person dies quietly at home. And because people experience a loved one's death privately, one family at a time, end-of-life care is especially different for health consumers, who often do not even know that the hospice option is available to them.

The result is that hospice is sorely underused. The need is growing; financial pressures from the status quo are mounting. That ought to foster a booming increase in hospice care rather than a modest decline. Why is this happening?

- Until the 1980s Medicare—the nation's largest health-insurance program—did not pay hospice organizations for providing care. Even now much of the cost of care is not reimbursed.

- Only a fraction of U.S. hospitals have staff trained to identify patients who are candidates for hospice and to help families tap that resource.

- Hospices struggle to provide care to people who live in nursing homes, because of turf and funding issues.

- Medicare's eligibility rules discourage doctors from considering hospice as an option for their dying patients. For people with kidney failure to qualify for hospice, for example, they must cease dialysis—even though that ensures their death from blood poisoning in weeks if not days.

The same is true of all curative treatment; for Medicare to pay a person's hospice bills, the patient must effectively stop seeking a cure. In other words, the patient must choose between living as long as possible or as well as possible. Government policy does not allow someone to pursue both.

Here's a grim example of eligibility rules that chill hospice use: The physician must provide a signed certification that the patient will be dead within six months. In addition to heartlessness, the problems with that policy are many. First, studies have found that doctors are notoriously bad at predicting when patients will die. Second, if a doctor's patients outlive the prediction, the physician may be prosecuted for Medicare fraud. No wonder doctors resist directing patients to hospice. No wonder a growing number of hospice patients enter its home-care program only days before dying.

But the worst aspect of this eligibility rule is the effect it has on patients and their families. Because of the six-month certification requirement, patients equate entering hospice with surrendering the fight to stay alive. Families consider the suggestion of hospice a sign that the doctor has given up.

Add these forces together and the result is clear: While seven-eighths of the population want to die at home, without needless suffering, less than one-fifth actually does so. All the positive attributes of hospice are not enough to make it popular.

·   ·   ·

NOT SURPRISINGLY, there is a growing effort to bring some hospice principles into hospitals, by providing what is known as "palliative care." In general, to palliate means to reduce the violence of something, to mitigate or soften its negatives. In gradual dying there inevitably comes a point when patients are not ever going to get better. But the fact that they cannot be cured does not mean that the tools and techniques of medicine cannot make their remaining life much better, that the negatives cannot be softened.

Consider a palliative approach to a woman with advanced lung cancer. After months or years of her battling the disease, it has finally spread throughout her body. She is not going to recover. She may have months before the cancer takes her life, but one morning she has difficulty breathing. She experiences panic and desperate coughing. Her oncologist finds a tumor in her esophagus. He promptly orders radiation therapy on that tumor. This treatment will not stop the disease, but it will prevent future episodes of compromised breathing. The patient will still die of lung cancer, but she will not gasp and choke in her remaining months, nor suffocate prematurely because of a preventable blockage. Her treatment has been palliative, providing not a cure but comfort.

Palliative care is important for many reasons. First, there will always be patients who feel more secure within a health-care institution, people for whom the size and resources of a hospital are reassuring. A preference so central to their emotional well-being merits respect. Second, physicians observing the shift toward gradual dying may find it easier to advocate for better care within existing facilities than to create new programs. Third, palliative care's attention to comfort is applicable to many patients beyond those whose death is imminent.

"We're working way upstream of hospice," says Diane Meier, M.D., who runs the palliative-care program at Mount Sinai Hospital in New York City. "From the moment you are diagnosed you receive both life-prolonging therapy and palliative care, until the very end when the patient is no longer able to benefit from the life-prolonging work, at which point care should focus one hundred percent on palliative care."

Like many hospice advocates, Meier partly defines her work by what it is not. "Palliative care is not about convincing people that it's okay to die. Palliative care is about helping people achieve the best quality of life they possibly can, for as long as they possibly can."

Finding demand for palliative care is not an issue, Meier says. When

Mount Sinai started its program in 1997, "we expected fifty patients that year. We had two hundred and fifty. Last year we had nine hundred new patient consults, and we've had roughly five thousand patient visits since 'ninety-seven."

Doctors who direct patients to palliative care often become allies, because it lessens their workload. "You take a doctor, an oncologist, say, and he's got forty patients in his waiting room. He cannot spend an hour in a family meeting, discussing issues and options. We can. We do."

In addition to her medical duties, Meier is an advocate. She directs the Center to Advance Palliative Care, which works to spread palliative care around the country.

"We provide technical assistance to local leaders on how to make the business case," Meier says, "how to project the need and the value of palliative care, how to measure your work to ensure quality, how to bill, how to launch a program that actually delivers on what it promises."

From a technical standpoint, palliative care is not difficult to provide, Meier says, yet most doctors don't know how. Persuading cash-strapped hospital administrators to undergo the expense of teaching them—and then to adopt palliative care principles permanently—is a real challenge.

"Doctors don't know how to do this stuff, it's so arcane. There is plenty of content available on how to manage pain, but it is not enough to get the care to the bedside. You have to justify your existence."

Yet hospitals have many reasons to provide palliative care, Meier says. "There is both conclusive data and widespread public awareness that patients are suffering. And the business argument for change is also powerful. Hospitals with a growing population of increasingly frail patients are not going to make it without a palliative-care approach."

Meier is quick to boast that the number of hospitals moving into palliative care is fast growing, nearing 20 percent. Those inroads have resulted in part from the success of palliative care in hospitals that have embraced it, and in fair measure because of $23 million in Robert Wood Johnson Foundation funding for the advocacy center Meier runs. Despite all that spending and the clear need for improved care, however, 80 percent of U.S. hospitals have not embraced a commitment to ensuring patients' comfort at the end of their lives. Like hospice, palliative care has a long way to go.

It is fair to ask, too, why a matter as important as patients' comfort should be shuttled off to a distinct service within a hospital. Why should regular medicine shrug off these responsibilities? The job of compassionate patient care needs to be done everywhere, just as every doctor and nurse needs to know how to take vital signs. If something affects 100 percent of patients, shouldn't at least its rudiments be known by 100 percent of practitioners, with expertise available in 100 percent of institutions? The lessons of empathy and listening, of responding to patient needs, are valuable not only in terminal care. Virtually every aspect of contemporary medicine could benefit from greater humanism and heart.

SOME OF THE MOST TROUBLING DATA about end-of-life care comes from the Center for Evaluative Clinical Sciences at Dartmouth Medical College. Director John Wennberg, M.D., has made a career of digging through the records of Americans' use of health services. His work stems from the reasonable premise that spending more on treatment makes sense only if you get better results. Over and over, he has found, that logic is reversed. He has discovered huge variations between one region of the country and another in the quantity of care doctors and hospitals deliver, with no correlating difference in people's health.

Wennberg's end-of-life-care data fit the pattern. In one part of the country about one-sixth of dying patients wound up in the hospital. In other areas the number was more than half. In some places one in twelve people died in an ICU; in other regions one in three. People in some parts of the country saw a doctor nine times in the last six months of life; in others, visits to physicians neared fifty. The number of patients seeing more than ten doctors in their final six months of life ranged from 3 percent in some regions to 30 percent elsewhere.

The most striking gap was financial. In some parts of the country average Medicare spending per terminal patient was $6,200. In other areas the spending was $18,000, nearly triple.

Quite apart from the financial impact, it is easy to imagine the different experiences dying people would have in each of these places: the stress of getting to five times as many doctor appointments, the doubled drama of twice as much intensive care, and so on.

Wennberg's research contains two stunning findings. First, higher spending does not result in longer lives or better deaths. "Populations living in regions with lower intensity care in the last six months of life did not have higher mortality rates," he writes in the *Dartmouth Atlas of Health Care*.

Think of it: Even in places with triple the spending, the mortality rate is no better.

Second, the rate at which a region spends money on terminal patients is not determined by the intensity of efforts to lengthen life or improve care. Instead, it is primarily "influenced by the available supply of acute care hospital resources." Spending is not based on patient needs, he concludes, but on the supply of equipment and facilities.

Wennberg's data raises a host of medical and ethical questions. Is the health system self-serving rather than patient-serving? Are some people receiving too much care, at public expense, while others receive too little? How are these literally life-and-death decisions being made, and by whom?

Lacking concrete answers to these questions, Wennberg's research may reveal something more human. Call it a searching—a costly, fumbling attempt to help people die as they deserve. Maybe, as his study implies, the search is driven by money. Or perhaps the motives are less cynical. Maybe the health system wants to help but doesn't know how. So we build a hospital, add intensive-care beds, and hope it makes a difference. After all, this approach worked wonderfully for heart attacks. Shouldn't it work for the growing list of incremental illnesses?

All the data says that it has not. America needs a different model. Now that most people die gradually, it is time for a new approach.

Ironically, one of the main obstacles is the effect of good intentions. When doctors see illness, they are conditioned by training, experience, and personal inclination to take action. They have no time to sit with a patient, simply sit, providing nothing more and nothing less than human presence. The treatments doctors offer, the tests they order, provide distraction and maybe shallow comfort. But when a patient is irreversibly dying, doctors' heroic interventions are like the proverb of the man with only a hammer, who sees every problem as a nail.

Families' good intentions add to the emotional tangle. Too often family members are not ready to lose the people they love, so they subject parents or spouses to all manner of undignified ordeals. Other times families pursue heroic measures beyond the point of futility, not because they expect the patient to improve but because they have confused medical persistence with genuine devotion.

Patients themselves are not exempt from well-meaning motives that complicate end-of-life care. For some, another surgery buys time in which a child or spouse can prepare for the loss to come. For others, the idea of being a burden on the healthy is so repugnant that they insist on suffering needlessly. Either way, patients miss the rich opportunity gradual dying provides, not realizing what has passed them by—though they get only one death, only one time to do it right.

It may sound bizarre, but it is true: There is such a thing as a beautiful death. That is not Pollyanna thinking; it is the promise and the potential made possible by gradual dying. There is such a thing as a beautiful death.

SHIFTING HEALTH CARE to accommodate today's manner of dying may sound like a daunting task. But there is a role model, in the changes in emergency care that saved Jack's life. Institutional medicine has played a modest role. Far larger has been the influence of health consumers, who insisted on emergency services that reflected their genuine needs and who learned how to participate in their care and that of people they love.

The needs for end-of-life care are analogous: Just as 911 phone service activates emergency medicine, America needs to establish a responsive system for summoning excellent end-of-life care. In the same way that a half-day CPR course prepares ordinary people to help others avoid sudden death, America needs a class that teaches people how to seize the opportunity presented by slow dying.

Given this analogy, there are two encouraging factors in end-of-life care. First, unlike emergency medicine, decent treatment for dying people is relatively inexpensive. Rather than revolving around doctors, it relies on nurses, volunteers, and families to provide care. Instead of powerful drugs that restart hearts and open clogged arteries, it requires common pain medicines. Compassionate end-of-life care minimizes recourse to costly surgeries or heroic technologies. And it uses patients' own homes rather than hospitals' expensive trauma-care beds.

Second, emergency medicine is complex, requiring advanced diagnostic tools and personnel with special training. Proper end-of-life care is often simple, from a medical standpoint, and the paramount job qualification is empathy.

When it comes to dying, American society today is like a subterranean explorer trying to find his way out of a cave. First we must light the inner cavern, so we know where we are. Then we need to illuminate the winding paths ahead, to find our way to daylight and fresh air.

CHAPTER FIVE

SO MUCH POTENTIAL

When people we love die, regardless of our religious faith, we gain comfort in the belief that their energy persists in this world. The work they did remains. The people they loved carry memories. Their children walk the earth. The force of their being is reaffirmed every time somebody misses them or sees them in a dream or performs some action solely because the deceased one would have appreciated it.

These are ripples in the waters of existence, signs that we endure beyond the moment when our breath stops, evidence of life's power to absorb death and surpass it.

This force is much larger, though, than a person's idiosyncrasies, habits, generosities, and mistakes. It is nearer to the Buddhist notion of interconnectedness, which sees all things in creation as linked and therefore considers one life, one small human life amid the infinite universe, as nonetheless cosmic in its consequences.

The same resonance exists when it comes to a person's passage from this life into whatever awaits. The manner of a death has greatest import to the person whose life is ending, of course, who either suffers or achieves peace, frets or finds calm. But the meaning of a death also matters long afterward to people close to the deceased. Most people's feelings of grief and loss eventually ease, because time is merciful. But other emotions persist. If the patient's death went badly, after grief fades there may be lingering guilt and regret, and these feelings can be lifelong. Conversely, if a death goes well, once the survivors heal their grief they discover an enduring sense of satisfaction, from helping someone they loved achieve a dignified end on his or her own terms. This feeling lasts the rest of their lives.

The point is that a death causes ripples every bit as much as a life. This is the true imprint a body makes—not merely an outline in the snow, but an enduring shape in the world.

Never before, though, has humanity possessed greater powers to influence the manner of death. Never have there been better diagnostic tools to make diseases' paths predictable. Never superior medicines for the treatment of pain. Never a population more determined to shape its destiny whenever possible.

Think of it: You can help the people you love die with dignity and fulfillment. You have the potential to experience the enduring gratification of this profoundly compassionate work. You also have the capacity to ensure deliverance for yourself, to make your life's last months and weeks as meaningful and resonant as your best days of health and action and glory.

Whether on behalf of your father or mother, your lover, or yourself, here is a moment worthy of preparation. The interval between when you know for certain that a death is coming and the instant when it actually arrives may be the most important time in your life.

PART TWO

NOT AN EMERGENCY

THE SWAN

*This laboring through what is still undone,
as though, legs bound, we hobbled along the way,
is like the awkward walking of the swan.*

*And dying—to let go, no longer feel
the solid ground we stand on every day—
is like his anxious letting himself fall*

*into the water, which receives him gently
and which, as though with reverence and joy,
draws back past him in streams on either side;
while, infinitely silent and aware,
in his full majesty and ever more
indifferent, he condescends to glide.*

—RAINER MARIA RILKE

CHAPTER SIX

WHAT IS A CRISIS?

Suppose you were confronted with a dead body: a coworker slumped at his desk, a stranger motionless on the sidewalk, a loved one whose life completed hours before you arrived home at the end of the day. Of course, you would first assure yourself that the life spirit was truly, irrevocably gone. But then, presuming the person was genuinely dead, with no chance of reawakening, would you know what to do?

Probably not. That's one sure sign of how unfamiliar death has become. For virtually all of human history people experienced dying at close range. They watched it occur, participated in preparing the body, constructed the coffin, dug the grave or built the pyre. If a person performed these tasks today, far from being perceived as devoted, he or she might well be considered ghoulish. Touching the corpse, even of a beloved, is taboo. A dead body is so alien in contemporary America that few people outside the medical field know what to do when they encounter one. From this unintentional ignorance, it is a long journey to treating a dying person with reverence.

Many people would dial 911. Certainly if there is any hope for the person to survive, the call makes sense. But if your boss has been bent over his desk for so long that he's gone cold, or the sidewalk stranger has no breath or pulse whatsoever, or your grandmother at day's end sits rigidly beside her untouched breakfast, there is no emergency.

Yet upon seeing a dead body, many Americans treat it as an urgent situation. It's an understandable reaction. They have no idea what to do. They are probably afraid. No one has told them what happens when a person dies. They panic. They call for help.

It may not be the help they bargained for. Emergency squads do not treat a dead body as dead. After several pertinent court cases, especially an influential 1998 decision by the Massachusetts Supreme Court, in all but the most extreme and gruesome cases EMTs are not permitted to declare a person dead. Only a physician can do that. So the technicians use all their tools—scissoring away clothes, shocking the heart, injecting adrenaline—on a corpse. They load the body on a stretcher and cart it off to a hospital, knowing the prognosis well in advance.

If you try to intervene, you will quickly discover that courts have limited your authority to do so. You do not get a vote. If you say, "But he's already dead" or "Why are you pounding on Grandma's chest?" the EMTs will politely ask you to step aside. The body is not your property. Legally, the case can be made, it is theirs. And in their domain it will remain, their responsibility, unless you can instantly produce documents proving that you have medical power of attorney. Anything less and you are only interfering.

This situation is not the fault of EMTs, who routinely save the lives of people in situations of medical trauma or crisis. Their training is to do all they can. Their concern, too, is avoiding a lawsuit for failing to do anything less. If you persist in trying to stop treatment, the rescue squad's response will soon stop being polite.

Then off they race, body in the back, sirens blaring, while you try to decide what to do first—call a friend, hire a lawyer, or follow the ambulance on your own.

What is a crisis? A car accident. A sudden fall. A heart attack or stroke. An urgent situation in which a person needs medical attention right away.

What is not a crisis? The gradual process of a body succumbing to an incremental disease. A situation in which medical treatment is futile.

Not only are Americans unschooled in death in general, they are particularly unprepared for its new, gradual manifestation. They look away in sadness and fear, but they see the same incremental, relentless illness when they glance back. It is tragedy in slow motion.

The result in many cases is anguish while the person is dying, and self-doubt or guilt long after the person is gone. People know a friend is nearing death, but they don't call or visit for fear of interfering. Families leave medical decisions to overburdened health professionals instead of providing comfort themselves. Coworkers, bowling buddies, church friends, and golf partners all withdraw because they don't want to impose.

They're quick to send flowers afterward, but that does the dying person little good.

These people are no more to blame than the EMTs, really. Until they learn how gradual dying happens, the actual events and likely sequence, they are treading on foreign ground.

WHAT OCCURS AFTER DEATH is an unknown; the process of dying gradually is not. Demystifying incremental death can enable people to face it with greater courage. A person who knows what to expect and has time to consider how to act is later freed of echoing questions or self-recrimination. When the end of life is less alien, compassion can overcome fear.

As dying has become gradual, it has also become predictable. Of course, each person with a terminal illness is unique, and the pace of the disease will likewise be individualistic. Nevertheless, there is a course that dying follows. It is knowable. Thus, its power to instill panic, to compound grief by adding fear, can be profoundly diminished if people only know what is happening, why, and, most crucially, what can be done.

At first, looking directly at death may not seem easy. But in reality it is a fascinating and enlightening process, life's ultimate mystery and only certainty. Besides, until recently, dying was part of everyday life.

Historically "families bore the bulk of medical expenses," Joanne Lynn, M.D., writes in a Rand Corporation study, "and the main caregivers were family members, especially women—mothers, wives and daughters. People generally lived out their days at home among family members."

Not anymore. Intimate connections such as closing the eyes of a dead loved one are beyond rare. Health insurance and Medicare pay much of the expenses. And the caregiving comes from well-meaning but total strangers who work in hospitals and nursing homes. Until their loved ones lie in the last light, families today do not know mortality.

That shift is ironic, given medical science's victories over the sudden causes of death. Think of it this way: Would you, if your mother were bedridden and weak and near the end, know how to turn her over in bed? It's an important skill to know, to keep her comfortable and to avoid bedsores. Yet accomplishing this task without hurting her or straining your back is more obscure to many people than knowing how their car's catalytic converter works. The larger point is this: At the moment that many

Americans might best improve the quality of their loved ones' final days, they are least equipped to do so.

There is a strong imperative for changing that situation. People who die slowly need help. They need someone to advocate for them, make medical decisions for them, read to them. They need someone to listen, wet their lips, hold their hand. None of these tasks is covered by health insurance, so few of them will be performed by medical professionals.

Dr. Lynn describes the situation in understated fashion: "As currently configured, health care and community services are not organized to meet the needs of the large and growing number of people facing a long period of progressive illness and disability before death."

"Not organized" is a polite way of saying ill-equipped and actually designed for the opposite purpose. A patient in crisis falls well within the expertise of contemporary American health care; a person dying by slow degrees does not. Therefore the burden of care, as more Americans' lives end gradually, increasingly falls to their families. History is repeating itself. This time, though, family members are unprepared for the responsibilities they will have to shoulder. It is time to begin to learn.

CHAPTER SEVEN

POSSIBLE PATHS

First we will discuss the common courses of dying today, then the patient's physical experience, then the emotional and spiritual one. Finally we will address some of the mysteries, the inexplicable things that can happen just before a person dies, and what they might mean.

HEALTH-POLICY EXPERTS refer to slow dying as succumbing to chronic illness, by which they mean incurable health problems that worsen over a span of time. A broken leg heals; a faulty gallbladder can be removed. These are temporary problems, whereas terminal chronic illnesses, once they have afflicted the patient, never go away. Yes, multiple sclerosis can go into remission, Alzheimer's disease may progress slowly for a time, and some cancers can be repressed for so many years that the patient ultimately dies of something else altogether.

That said, a man with Parkinson's disease is not going to be free of it. A woman with Lou Gehrig's disease will never get better. AIDS, so far, can be managed but not cured.

Chronic illnesses like these are taking a growing portion of lives in America today. Back in 1965 physicians and researchers described the experience of a dying person as a "trajectory"—that is, the path one's health status follows over time. These trajectories can be drawn; although the graphs are extreme simplifications of complex situations, they nonetheless articulate how dying has changed in recent years.

Consider first the person who dies suddenly, of a heart attack, stroke, or accident. Their experience probably looks something like Figure 1:

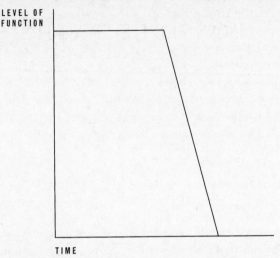

After the initial emergency effort, medical treatment of a person in this situation is minimal. The patient's family will need help dealing with shock and grief, but the caretaking does not involve the victim.

This kind of dying is less frequent with each passing year. In its place are myriad incremental illnesses that take lives slowly. Many follow paths that are not linear but are nonetheless predictable. Consider the experience of a cancer patient in Figure 2:

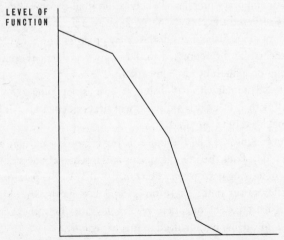

This trajectory of illness involves an initial period of high anxiety but high function. Any person diagnosed with cancer knows that it could be fatal; this person also knows that compromised energy and function will not be immediate. The patient may undergo major medical interventions—surgery, chemotherapy, and radiation. These efforts are so aggressive, it is possible to confuse their effects with those of the disease. But it is not cancer that makes a person's hair fall out, it is chemo. It is not cancer that is exhausting, at least in the early phases, but the radiation. By these means the progress of the disease may be slowed or even stopped. But then the cancer returns, invading more essential organs such as the liver, lungs, or brain. The patient begins a period of decline in function that this time is not due to treatment but to the disease. The final stage may come rapidly or decelerate to a merciless slowness, a lingering denouement that seems particularly cruel after what may have been years of living productively with the illness.

Overall, this trajectory challenges people who are ill by giving them a long-term fear of their future. The body can seem an alien thing, possessed by some external malice that somehow has become internal.

Conversely, people who have survived cancer often say the experience clarified their values, helped them shift priorities, and reminded them of the value of daily life. And even people who do not surmount their illness often enjoy months or years of high function, albeit with an ever present worry over what lies ahead.

This path challenges patients' families, too, because they live with many similar fears. They may also become accustomed to the disease's slow initial progress and be buoyed by its cycles so that its final effect leaves them feeling cheated. Most of all, they witness the decay of someone they love, the physical dwindling, fatigue, and weight loss, always with the understanding of where it will all end.

This path can be toughest for patients when the illness diminishes physical function but not mental acuity. Lou Gehrig's disease, for example, gradually suffocates the patient in a body incapacitated by the disease—yet the person's mind comprehends events until the last.

By contrast, Alzheimer's disease is emotionally gentler on the patient but harder for the family. The body is as vital as ever, but the personality slowly fades. By all manifestations, patients have little or no awareness of their predicament. That ignorance may be a mercy. However, as a patient reverts into a childlike state, albeit with all the physical demands of a healthy adult, caregivers can feel acutely lonely.

What this family may need more than medical interventions is respite care—small breaks to reengage with the functioning world and recharge the capacity to help patiently and with no expectation of thanks.

The emotions at the end of these illness paths may be difficult for families to acknowledge: relief, liberation, a sense of mercy that the struggle is over. The grieving commences long before anyone has died.

Yet not all the news in this trajectory is grim. Families whose loved ones contract these slow illnesses have the precious luxury of time. They have an opportunity to fulfill long-standing wishes, to mend fences, to provide loving care. Their task is hard but also potentially enriching.

A third common trajectory is what might previously have been called "old age," though medicine has dramatically changed what the phrase means. While people in this situation see their function and energy decay, death is not perceived as imminent. Their path is represented by Figure 3:

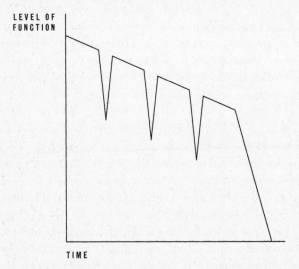

These people have a fair degree of function, with intermittent episodes of illness from which they always seem to recover. Hospitalizations with strong interventions bring consistently good results. This might be the path of people with lung disease who develop pneumonia, for example, are hospitalized for treatment, and bounce back. They go home not quite as spry as before but still with a high degree of function. They might have a knee problem, a digestive blockage, or a fall. But they reliably recover.

The challenges in this trajectory are no less serious. Foremost, the patient and family develop a belief that medical science can do anything, that every setback is surmountable if only the right steps are taken. Some of these patients boast about how many of their doctors they have outlived. Families say things like, "Grandma will be home soon, because that tough old goat has beaten six other problems in the past decade."

Neither health institutions nor medical-insurance programs are designed to reckon well with such cases. It is obviously difficult to predict which incident will be the one that initiates the final course, and thus satisfies Medicare's hospice requirement that a doctor certify that death will occur within six months. No one would want to prepare for Grandma to die if she actually has years of life remaining. So, when the final stage of her life does arrive, neither she nor her family recognizes what is happening. The temptation to deploy an arsenal of medical armaments could easily lead to the kind of dying few people would choose—in intensive care, sustained by machinery, at huge expense, and with little personalized treatment.

Only attentive and responsive doctors will know when to intercede, to win this patient a quiet death at home. Only the most realistically prepared and emotionally nimble of families will be ready, after so many successes, to accept medicine's limits and give her a dignified final experience.

THE SLOW-ILLNESS TRAJECTORIES share a common element that bears immediate mention: Whether the end comes from cancer, lung failure, or dementia (allowing for patients' varied constitutions) their final stages are nearly identical. When a person takes to his or her bed, the serious decline has begun. As body systems shut down, professional caregivers say the person is "actively dying." When a person stops taking fluids, he or she is days away from death. The last phase is now a predictable thing.

That foreknowledge is unprecedented in human history. The dying person knows roughly how much time is left. Families and friends know approximately when good-bye will come. The question is what people make of this knowledge. The ability to anticipate life's end could be as terrifying as a condemned man's walk to the gallows, or as liberating as a bird's taking flight. There is more than one path.

·　　·　　·

WHAT HAPPENS WHEN A PERSON DIES? At the most basic level, the body completes a natural process of shutting down, of discontinuing its life-sustaining systems. Dying is the means to that end, the step-by-step succumbing. Setting aside for a moment the emotional and spiritual aspects of this process, profound as they are, on a purely physical level the final changes are actually quite orderly. There is a natural, even normal, way that the body prepares itself to stop. Therefore, there are opportunities for people to participate, easing this process for someone they love.

It bears repeating that every person is unique. Just as no two lives are the same, neither are any two deaths. Health-care professionals who have witnessed many deaths say that people's manner of dying often mirrors their lives. Thus, the following physical stages may occur in a different order, and at a different pace. But knowing the range of what to expect can help everyone involved.

As a body shuts down, the circulation of blood weakens, concentrating in the most essential organs. As a result, a dying person's hands will one day feel cool to the touch. The process will later include the arms, feet, and legs. Skin color may lose its ruddy glow.

The experience for families and friends observing this shift can be painful. They arrive for a visit, squeeze their loved one's hand, and feel a chilly premonition of death. They look down to see fingernails turned blue. The challenge right then is to resist the impulse to withdraw. The patient only wants what anyone with cold hands wants: to be made warm.

This is one small example of how a little foreknowledge and a little courage can dramatically affect the quality of the experience for everyone involved. People who don't know that the moment of cold hands is coming will be surprised by it. They may pull back, leaving the patient feeling isolated and ashamed of dying. If people have been taught about the process of dying, though, they will be prepared. They will clasp the patient's hands in their own, warm them with their breath, add another blanket to the bedding. They will also know, sadly enough, that these hands are never going to be warm again. But that makes providing comfort all the sweeter.

Pain control is a central end-of-life challenge. Terminal illnesses vary widely in how much pain patients experience. The drug options for controlling pain have made huge strides in recent years, however, and nearly all patients' pain can be managed. Many doctors are reluctant to prescribe pain medication aggressively, so families bear responsibility for advocating on a patient's behalf. Once that job is done, the greater challenge is balancing pain treatment with a patient's desire to be awake. The dose of morphine that quiets aching bone cancer may also silence conversation. A visit during soporific times can be frustrating for both the patient and his visitors. The good news is that medical understanding of pain, and the array of treatment options, has never been better. A well-timed stimulant can keep a patient alert, for example, without diminishing pain management. Likewise, treating pain before it becomes severe, through what is called preemptive analgesia, frequently reduces the amount of pain medication the patient needs.

Some people believe they must suffer while dying. That attitude is a challenge for their caregivers. From a practical standpoint, though, there is simply no reason for a person to experience unwanted physical pain at the end of life. No patient should accept it. No family should allow it.

Once a terminal illness is in its most advanced stage, treating pain may have the side effect of making patients weary. Inevitably, whether from medication or illness, the time will come when they spend most of the day sleeping. During waking hours, concentration demands more effort. Communication becomes simpler, shorter, and rarer. Patients need help eating, drinking, and turning in bed. In this vulnerability and dependency, a kind of second infancy occurs. This period can possess an unexpected grace, allowing for special tenderness. Everyone sees that gradual dying is neither frantic nor fearful. It approaches slowly, peacefully.

One of the more challenging stages at this point is the loss of bladder and bowel control. For caretakers, incontinence means unpleasant tasks. For patients, it means lost dignity. After a lifetime of adult function, someone must help them pee, someone must wipe their bottom.

This stage is a good time to involve a nurse or aide—not simply to do the dirty work but to teach you how to minimize the mess and to respect everyone's dignity. A catheter may solve the problem simply. An aide or hospice volunteer may help bathe the person who is ill. People lovingly change a child's diaper at the start of life; they can lovingly perform similar tasks at the end of life.

The challenge is primarily to meet the emotional needs of patients, by preserving their dignity. But this effort also benefits caregivers. Families grieve differently, and often less, when they have the balancing emotions of gratification from doing a difficult job well. Medical professionals who concentrate on end-of-life care also stand tall when they talk of the work's emotional rewards.

Ira Byock, M.D., an end-of-life care expert and author, recalled treating a former politician who was terminally ill and whose dignity was wounded by an embarrassing bowel problem.

"Interactions just like this, caring and being cared for, are the way in which community is created," Byock told the man. "I believe that the word *community,* like the word *family,* is really more of a verb than a noun. Community comes about in the process of caring for those in need among us. It's unfortunate that now you're getting to see that side of it, but in allowing yourself to be cared for and being a willing recipient of care, you're contributing in a remarkably valuable way to the community. In a real sense, we need to care for you."

In other words, allowing care sends out ripples of tenderness. There is a great deal of dignity for a patient who has that effect on other people.

In terms of the physical process, the next phase may render incontinence issues moot: the loss of appetite. As a body concentrates its remaining powers on essential tasks like breathing and blood circulation, digesting becomes too much work. Patients stop feeding themselves. When a spoon is raised to their lips, they will turn their face away.

This is another instance in which families and medical caregivers may discover the conflicts resulting from good intentions. Studies by Roeline Pasman, Ph.D., investigated whether to force-feed nursing-home patients who have advanced dementia. Do patients turn their head away because they do not want food, or because they no longer know what it is?

These questions often land at the feet of spouses, siblings, or children. "The family has to be prepared for the death, and the possible decisions that may have to be made," Pasman writes.

Families are not alone in this dilemma. Diminished appetite can "cause a lot of stress and uncertainty, especially among the nursing staff. They experience a bad food- and fluid-intake of the patient as their problem and their shortcoming, instead of a process inherent to the illness trajectory."

Who should determine whether or not to continue feeding and how to make this wrenching decision are questions addressed later. For now, suffice it to say that all patients dying of incremental illness, regardless of the resolve of nurses, family members, and friends, eventually stop eating. Their fluid intake, too, may drop to almost nothing.

Determining the wishes of patients entering this phase of the dying process can be difficult, because they may have become uncommunicative. Too few people establish in advance what they would prefer. Pasman developed a set of external indicators—facial expressions, body tension, fidgeting, and noisy breathing—and applied them to 178 nursing-home patients with dementia who had stopping eating and drinking. The lack of sustaining nutrition did not prove to cause "high levels of discomfort, and therefore seems to be an acceptable decision."

Pasman's findings echo those reported in many U.S. medical journals. For example, one study asked nurses who care for the terminally ill to rate the quality of the death of patients who stopped eating and drinking. Given a scale of 0–9, with 0 meaning very bad and 9 being very good, the nurses gave their patients a median score of 8. The dying people experienced only the limited discomfort of a dry mouth.

At a minimum, therefore, caregivers should be ready with ice chips and glycerin lip swabs. There is more to be done, though; Pasman also found that treating patients' other symptoms—breathing difficulties, for example—remained an issue after eating and drinking had stopped. And in nursing homes, which frequently employ too few workers with medical training, attention to those symptoms is inconsistent at best.

Thus, patients who stop eating still need someone to advocate on their behalf for proper symptom management, for pain relief and oxygen support and medications to prevent seizures. But that illustrates how attending to comfort can be superior to intervening more aggressively: Obtaining things like proper pain medication will accomplish far more for the patient's benefit than wedging one more spoonful of pureed prunes between resistant lips.

What can families and friends expect when this phase arrives? A person who stops eating usually remains alive another two weeks or so. If someone stops taking fluids, the time is roughly halved.

In the last day or two, the person dying gradually will breathe differently. Respiration can become shallower and faster, sometimes even resembling gasps. This is not air hunger, as troubled bystanders might assume. Morphine, while controlling the patient's distress, is also decreasing sensation, so the lungs work as though they are deprived. People in this phase sometimes gurgle as they breathe, and the noise can be harder on bedside family members than for the patient. It sounds almost like drowning, though the actual cause is just a thin membrane of fluid near the vocal cords.

Eventually the patient breathes ever more slowly. This shift is a signal that circulation is decreasing in the respiratory center of the nervous system. Sometimes it may seem as though breathing has stopped completely, until a few deep sighs restart the rhythm. Now the end is quite near.

Doctors and nurses often say that hearing is the last external function to go. What a potential blessing this can be, with a little imagination. Might the dying person like to hear a favorite story retold? Or prefer to hear a beloved grandchild's voice one last time? What music—whether Beethoven or Springsteen, Benny Goodman or Bob Dylan—befits the last sensations of this person on earth?

There is one other merciful aspect in gradual dying that many clinicians attest to. Dying in this way—slowly, one step at a time—is gentle. When circulation and blood-oxygen levels are reduced, the extremities' messages of pain are muted. When mental functions are circumscribed to managing breath and heartbeat, awareness of life's imminent end is blunted. Sensations and thoughts become distant and mild. When fatigue overcomes the body, nothing is more appealing than rest.

This is the humane possibility inherent in gradual dying. On that path almost all people die in their sleep.

CHAPTER EIGHT

STILL ALIVE

To understand how the emotional process of dying differs from the physical one, only consider pain.

A man with terminal colon cancer has acute body discomfort, which narcotics can vanquish. The same man, with an estranged son, endures a kind of suffering that is far less easily assuaged.

The physical process of dying is largely a medical event, with symptoms, tests, procedures, and medicines. It is fundamentally a story about a *disease*. The emotional process of dying is almost wholly nonmedical, pertaining to incorporeal concerns. It is fundamentally a story about a *person*.

Because knowledge of the predictable physical steps can be useful in a patient's care, it is worth asking: To what extent can the mental, spiritual, and emotional aspects also be foreseen?

Any answer to this question must begin with Elisabeth Kübler-Ross, M.D. Forty years ago this Swiss physician broke the powerful taboo around death in America by interviewing thousands of dying people. She called terminal patients her "teachers" and published groundbreaking books on the emotional condition of people in the final phase of their lives. Distilled, Kübler-Ross's findings show that grief occurs in five identifiable stages: denial, anger, bargaining, depression, and acceptance.

All these reactions are familiar to doctors who treat people with terminal illness: "No, no, I can't possibly have cancer." "You damn doctors don't know what you're doing." "Dear God, let me live and I will dedicate my life to good works." "Maybe I should commit suicide now and avoid all the pain and suffering ahead." And finally: "Doctor, tell me what dying is like."

Families also follow Kübler-Ross's pattern. They shift from phase to phase, sometimes changing within a single sentence of conversation. And no wonder. They are wrestling with the ultimate metaphysical question, as well as sadness and feelings of loss, compounded by the responsibility of making complex medical decisions.

Hospice nurses Maggie Callanan and Patricia Kelley capture these phases, and how patients and families move through them, in an anecdote from their book *Final Gifts*.

Julia was finishing radiation for inoperable lung cancer when the doctor told her and her husband that she had about three months to live. Julia then informed her daughters, Jane and Sally, who lived in the area, and their son, John, on the West Coast. The hospice nurse arrived to find Jane weeping in the kitchen.

Jane's mother was insisting she'd be fine if she could only start eating again, which led Jane's father to leave the house in a rage. Jane's brother John was advocating for an experimental treatment, while her sister Sally was ready to make funeral arrangements.

Days later when the nurse returned, everyone's attitude had changed. Jane's parents had made funeral plans. Jane had blasted her father for his conduct. Sally was interested in the new medical idea and John was worried he might not get home before his mother died.

"In short order," Callanan and Kelley continue, "Jane had gone from depression to anger, Mom from denial to acceptance, Dad from anger to depression, Sally from acceptance to bargaining, and John from bargaining to depression, then acceptance."

It is tempting to think that each person—whether patient, friend, or family member—must move promptly to acceptance as a demonstration of emotional health. In fact, Kübler-Ross argued that much of the difficulty Americans have with death stems from society-wide denial of its existence.

A story from her early research gives that accusation teeth: Kübler-Ross went to a hospital and asked the unit manager if she could speak with the patients who were dying. There are none on this ward, she was told, so Kübler-Ross went to the next unit. The answer there was the same. She eventually canvassed the entire six-hundred-bed hospital, until there were no wards or floors left, and still no one was able to direct her to a dying patient.

Forty years after Kübler-Ross's first publications, the problem of denial has become common parlance. False optimism, like any faith grounded in untruth, ultimately damages the believer most. Disillusionment is certain to come, especially when the truth is as unavoidable as death. Indeed, greater realism might reduce the abandonment of people who are dying.

Beyond denial, it could be that Americans struggle with death because they have made nearly everything else in their lives subject to reason, systemization, and control—from the timing of conception and manner of birth onward. Only death remains outside the corral, the wild horse that will not be tamed.

In Kübler-Ross's lexicon, denial is an error and a sign of ill health. But there are dangers in ascribing universally negative connotations to people's emotional responses to dying. Each of the phases Kübler-Ross identified has a value that should not be ignored. Bargaining can be a way of rediscovering priorities and remembering what is important. Criticism of depression ignores the reality that mourning can be meaningful and that a person nearing life's end has ample reason to be sad. Denial can be close kin to persistence and optimism, inspiring people to explore all their clinical options—some of which may succeed. And anger? Maybe for a person who has been cheated, whose life has been unfair, reacting to a terminal diagnosis with anger is a mentally healthy response. An overwhelming emphasis on acceptance dismisses grief in a condescending manner. In all, who can judge what is emotionally appropriate for a person grappling with his life's end?

People who compel others to cease denial are committing the emotional equivalent of force-feeding, their good intentions inadvertently inflicting a cruelty. There is a risk of killing patients' hope at a time when it may be a key factor in the quality of their remaining life.

Hope. It is a perfect example of a nonmedical force that matters immensely. Researchers have repeatedly found evidence that patients' mental attitude can influence their susceptibility to illness, as well as a disease's course and speed. Moreover, some people are just plain happiest fighting to the bitter end.

"We are just beginning to appreciate hope's reach and have not defined its limits," writes Jerome Groopman, M.D.

"I see hope as the very heart of healing," he says. "For those who have hope, it may help some to live longer, and it will help all to live better."

·　　·　　·

THE POINT IS THAT the canon of thought on dying's emotional dimensions is subject to debate. That is especially so today, as more people have a slow approach to the end of their lives.

Let us draw an analogy, then. As discussed, there are three common trajectories for the physical process of gradual dying. Likewise there are a range of possible emotional journeys that patients and their loved ones may make. Just as the physical roads all lead to a similar final path, the emotional needs of dying people also converge in a common set of concerns.

Doctors and nurses say a sure sign of those needs is agitation. A person who is dying with unresolved worries will be restless, shifting in bed, repeating some insignificant task, reiterating some statement that may not make immediate sense.

Caregivers may see these actions as medical symptoms and call for sedatives. That could be a mistake. Drugs will silence the behavior but not the underlying emotions. The correct response may seem self-evident, but people in the midst of grief and fear do not always think clearly about what they ought to do: Ask what is wrong, and then listen.

Patients may have relationship conflicts they want to resolve. It's not always possible to accomplish, of course, but the quiet humility people feel beside a deathbed makes possible all manner of reconciliations. The patient may have spiritual questions; nearly all medical institutions have chaplains at the ready. The dying person may be afraid; an experienced nurse can describe the physical process in an unthreatening way. Patients may want to die in a certain location; often this desire is evidence of an effort to take care of the living even as they are dying.

There are common fears—of lingering in pain, of becoming too great a burden on the living, even of being buried alive. It is not difficult to reassure people about these concerns.

Patients may want some aspect of their life organized before they can be at peace; the tasks are typically small, more symbolic than substantial. Or they may be concerned about how a family member will manage without them; this need challenges people to provide their ailing loved ones with reassurance, giving them permission to die.

It is valuable to remember that talking to a person about dying does not cause it to occur. Likewise, crying in front of a person who is terminally ill generally reveals not weakness but affection. Ironically, the solemnity of dying can sometimes make patients crave humor, a little lightness, a break from the heavy work at hand.

Showing sincere emotion, in whatever form, can take courage. But families and friends who answer a dying loved one's needs experience a unique fulfillment. They make it possible for the person who is ill to relax, shun incidental concerns, and journey toward the unknown calmly. They have eased the way.

Sadly, their recompense sometimes comes in a cruel fashion: the person who is dying may withdraw from them. That same patient who counted on them every day for news and a hand massage now does not acknowledge when they enter the room. Families and friends in this situation can find themselves filled with self-doubt. Have they offended the sick person? What did they do wrong? No matter what they do, they find that the patient prefers to be with only a few select people, and they are not included.

People in this predicament need to know that they have done nothing wrong. On the contrary, decreased socialization by a person at the end of life signifies that emotionally, things are going well. Withdrawal does not mean that they have stopped loving anyone. It signifies that they have finished their business with that person. Like hands losing circulation as the body weakens physically, relationships become cool as the patient pares down to the one or two essential final caregivers. Being outside the inner circle is not rejection; it is affirmation that your work together is done.

It may seem obvious to say, but it is crucial to remember that people who are dying are not yet dead. They're still alive. That means they want all the normal things that any living being wants—warmth, companionship, emotional nourishment. At a time in human history when so many people face the journey out of life while feeling abandoned, families and friends can know that it is virtually impossible to err on the side of providing excessive care. Few people leave this world having experienced too much love.

CHAPTER NINE

MYSTERIES OF LIFE

Some aspects of the dying process defy explanation. Call them mysteries. They may not be explicable, but researchers have confirmed their occurrence time and again. These events are not occultish, nor do they contradict any religious faith. What they do, though, is suggest that death is a curtain through which it may be possible to peek. Above all, they reaffirm the vitality—the life force—still powerfully active in people even in their penultimate hours.

The most common of the mysteries is timing. People with terminal illness routinely outlive any reasonable prognosis, in order to witness a marriage, see a baby born, attend a graduation, reach some significant anniversary. Once the milestone is accomplished, life ends swiftly.

It even happens for people at the outermost precincts of consciousness. Although comatose, they soldier on while a sister flies across the country or a son drives from out of state. Once the missing person arrives, words are spoken, perhaps recognition attained, and the patient relinquishes his grip on existence. It happens with surprising frequency.

Doctors and nurses who provide care to terminal patients have also seen caretaking of the opposite sort. People who by all accounts should no longer be living manage to eke out hour upon inexplicable hour, until their spouse leaves to perform an errand. Then they die quickly. Did they intend to spare their loved one the experience of seeing them die?

Hospice nurses say this pattern is most acute when the patient is a child. Terminally ill youngsters can be surprisingly matter-of-fact about their situations. They manifest many behaviors that indicate they are trying to take care of their grieving parents. At the final stage, they often wait until Mom is fetching something from the car and Dad has gone to the coffee shop. It is uncanny: After prolonged parental vigilance, that solitary moment is the one in which the child dies.

Another common mystery occurs when people at the end of their lives appear to have visions. They converse with empty air. They talk about visitors, from previously deceased family members to angels to strangers who will guide them on the journey ahead.

Are these appearances evidence of life after death? Or are they delusions that the brain supplies itself, in order to quell the cognitive dissonance of knowing death is imminent? In a way, it doesn't matter. The important thing is that the person who is dying finds comfort in these visions. The healthy and living bystanders sometimes do, too.

From time to time nurses report that patients experiencing visions reveal information they have no reasonable means of possessing. A geographically distant uncle dies unexpectedly, and before anyone has brought the news, the dying person mentions having conversed with him. These situations occur often, and they are inexplicable.

Whole books have been written by physicians and scholars about the mysteries surrounding the time near death. The explanations range from the spiritual to the hard-to-swallow. Here they merit mention for two reasons, each a reason to regard dying with perhaps a little less fear.

First, these mysteries imply that the boundary between life and death is not sharp for people dying gradually. It is a blurry line, a transition zone. That mirrors the physical experience of a person whose breathing seems to stop, but who then sighs and continues. People near the end appear to go back and forth, showing not anxiety but ease, a welcoming of what is to come. Their actions suggest that the cessation of a life is not abrupt like a leap from a cliff, but incremental like swimming into deeper waters.

The second message of the mysteries is about strength. If dying patients see things a healthy person cannot, it implies that they are finding their own final comforts. If they can stretch their days to reach an important milestone, or hasten their end in order to lighten a loved one's grief, it implies that there is some kind of a life control within each of us, and the hand on that device is our own.

Think of it: The terminal cancer patient, the seemingly oblivious Alzheimer's victim, and the skeletal AIDS battler all have one thing in common. Even in what appears to be their weakest, most distressed state, they may still possess enormous power.

CHAPTER TEN

TWO VISIONS

When a person has died, there is no emergency. The most common signal of life's end is that breathing stops. With the end of an oxygen supply, the body's functions cease. The mouth may fall open slightly, the bladder release any inconsequential, last contents. There is no pulse at the neck or wrist, no thumping in the chest. As gravity makes blood pool, blue patches may appear on the underside of the body. Gradually the limbs cool, with the chest cavity remaining warm longest.

Grief is paramount at this moment, and the sole demand of that emotion is time. Haste often equates to hurt. There are no medical needs to be met. There may be needs for the family and friends, but the dead person requires nothing at all.

In time the sadness will quiet and there will be room for reflection. Then the central question is what people made of the caretaking opportunity that this person's gradual dying presented to them. Did they take good care of their loved one's physical requirements? Did they pay attention to emotional needs and respond to the ones that they could address? Did they strive to help the patient live well so that dying was only an instant that arrived after a loving, calm experience?

That is what people say they want. It is rarely what they achieve. Families may be tempted to blame themselves—as if they failed their loved one by not knowing in advance that dying has become gradual and by not advocating for dignified, personalized medical and emotional care. But it is not their fault. There are many impediments to their good intentions, obstacles no individual family has the power to surmount.

The greatest of these roadblocks is a health-care system that is organized to respond to death as it occurred a generation ago. Doctors are taught to treat diseases, not people. The delivery of health care, from staffing to billing, is organized around institutions instead of patients. Gradual dying is treated as a medical crisis instead of a natural process. The next chapter examines these obstacles, how they were constructed, and how they could be dismantled.

Here are two visions to keep in mind during that discussion. One is of an ambulance speeding down a road, lights flashing, siren wailing, while inside a dead body undergoes invasive and futile treatment.

The other is of a bedroom in a house in which a person has recently died. His hands are folded, hair combed, clothes straight, and blankets neatly arranged. Loved ones are gathered near, praying, crying, talking softly to one another, hugging and giving comfort. On the table a single candle is lit. And that room is so peaceful, the flame barely seems to flicker.

PART THREE

HEAL THYSELF

Let the beauty we love
be what we do.
There are a hundred ways
to kneel and kiss the ground.

—RUMI

CHAPTER ELEVEN

DOCTORS' BEGINNINGS

Abigail Donaldson of Lincoln, Massachusetts, cannot remember a time when she did not want to become a physician. Her father is a surgeon. Her brother is an internist. Abby followed a steady path, earning good grades year upon year, enduring the grueling admissions tests, working in research briefly, then entering medical school.

Nevertheless, she was anxious about her first day of gross anatomy. That semester-long lab, a medical school rite of passage, serves many purposes. It begins a student's indoctrination into the culture of a doctor's clinical relationship with a body. It provides early lessons in confidentiality about a patient's condition and history. As class partners take turns mastering certain subjects in order to make the group's memorization workload lighter, it delivers an unspoken introduction to the concepts of medical specialization and teamwork.

These are abstractions, though. In terms of the course content, gross anatomy is intended to acquaint young people like Abby with the concrete workings of the human machine. The lab involves complete dissection of a cadaver, from nose to toes, to teach shape and color and texture, and how it all fits together inside the tender vessel of skin. No piece is sacred—not the teeth, not the fingers, not the genitals. Manipulating the corpse releases the sharp pungency of its chemical preservatives, which clings to clothes and hair like the stink of skunk. Regardless, this is a time to learn—not through textbooks but by sight and touch—how the human organism is built. Exemplary structures are set aside for later class review. Aberrations uncovered during dissection are held up for all to see.

"I'd never seen a dead body before," Abby said. "Everyone in my family gets cremated. I was nervous. I was intimidated. I felt sort of unqualified to take apart this body that had encased a whole person. I'm this twenty-five-year-old who has taken one month of histology, and before that I was a history of science major. How is it that I am allowed to do this?"

Debate over direct anatomy instruction dates back centuries. Is cadaver study disrespectful of the human body, or reverent toward it? In the seventeenth century dissections were held publicly, crowds assembling to crack jokes during the procedure. A few decades ago medical students sometimes named the bodies they were disassembling, put hats or clothes on them, painted their fingernails. Some medical schools now substitute computers and 3-D lab results for whole-body dissection.

These schools are few, though, and ghoulish incidents increasingly rare. Most medical schools now insist upon respectful treatment of the cadaver. And most medical educators agree that direct experience with the body—actually touching the bones and vessels and organs—surpasses any other method of teaching fledgling physicians how the human machine works. Years later, doctors confronted with an unfamiliar illness will mentally picture the body parts involved, recalling how the pieces fit together. They say a pelvis is only an idea, a tidy illustration in a book, until you extract one from a body and feel its weight and strength in your hand. Nerves are yellow and delicate. The heart is surprisingly small.

Opening day of gross anatomy often marks the first time medical students have hands-on experience with death. They may have seen Grandma dressed nicely in her casket, or buried a goldfish in the backyard, but otherwise lifelessness stood at a considerable remove. Now, as they touch a naked corpse, slowly, deliberately, and completely, it is their initiation to the cold facts of mortality.

For Abby, the anticipation put her imagination to work. She wondered about the donors' families. "Do they realize what we're doing here? That we're exploring every nook and cranny, inside and out?"

She also could not help envisioning her cadaver's life. "This person was a member of the community. They could have children at my university; they could have grandchildren who run where I go."

The class was divided into teams of six for each body. Abby and her classmates readied themselves by purchasing basic surgical kits at the campus bookstore. Meanwhile, Abby couldn't stop wondering what her cadaver's face might look like. "I was worried about how I would react."

Finally on an autumn Monday afternoon she marched with her class-mates single file into the long lab room of covered stainless-steel tables. Beneath the metal hoods lay donated bodies, which arrive so swiftly after death that they often remain in whatever clothes the people were wearing when they drew their last breath. Medical schools' cadaver-donation man-agers report everything from shearing away old nightgowns to shredding business suits to scissoring off the life vest of a man who had drowned. The bodies receive "curatorial preservation" instead of regular embalming: no cosmetics, but more chemicals so the cadavers can lie out on a dis-secting table for four months without rotting. Prepared bodies then wait on racks in refrigerated rooms, all in anticipation of this moment.

The students gathered in their preselected groups at each station, where they were told how to work the table hood, where to place their in-struments, how to open the body bag.

"Students are mandated to carry out in the dissection lab a piecemeal dismemberment that would under any other circumstances be criminal or insane," write Kathy Johnson Neely, M.D., and Douglas Reifler, M.D., of Chicago. "And they are expected to accomplish it with little more emotion than distaste for the embalming fluid. Indeed for many students, the task of human dissection presents an 'emotional Rubicon' determining whether they have the right stuff to become a competent, unflappable physician."

When the time came, Abby and her classmates lifted the tabletops. The cadaver before her was as white as porcelain, with identifying num-bers inked in blue onto its arms. And the body was lying facedown.

"The head at that point was bagged," Abby remembered. "That made a big difference for me, that we didn't have to look at the face. That would force you to acknowledge that they're human. It was pretty impersonal, actually. You don't spend a lot of time looking at people's naked backs, but you see faces all day every day."

The team received basic information about its cadaver: female, age seventy-seven, dead of heart failure. Immediately Abby realized that her life had just begun a major shift. "We've all been in school; we're all good students. And lecture hall is just more of the same. But the anatomy lab, that is something few other people get to do. I'm no longer a student like every other kind of student. This is a different kind of school."

Abby's reverie was broken by instructions: She was told to make her first incision, in the lower spine. She hesitated.

"For me, that was the moment," Abby said. She took a deep breath. She coached herself. "I need to engage. I need to participate in the class and get over that hump. So I chiseled open the spine. The skin was thicker than I had expected it to be, cold and tough."

Instantly there was anatomical information to be memorized. In Latin.

"The first, preclinical years of medicine demand the student face an intense barrage of experiences with death," Neely and Reifler write. "The student typically responds by distancing him/herself."

Soon enough Abby found herself fascinated by the material. She discovered a distaste for fat and an appreciation for muscle. Gradually she understood that her chosen profession was different from anything else—the intimacy of it, the extent to which a doctor is entrusted. She felt conflicted, though, between immersing herself in the science and remembering that her instructional object had once been a person walking this earth.

"You could run the same class and have it be an emotional exploration of the human body," Abby said. "You know, what is your reaction to using handsaws and chisels and hammers on a human body? Fingernails—so what do you think about that? Taking skin off—it sticks in some places and not in others. What does that mean?"

But there is no time for such exploration. There is too much material to memorize. The shoulder socket alone is a byzantine maze of nerves, tendons, ligaments, and muscles, all wrapped together as densely as wires in the electric conduit of a skyscraper. Besides, the students hear repeatedly what an incredible privilege the dissection experience is.

It is a test, too, of students' capacity to set aside distaste in order to learn. At some medical schools, for example, when it is time to study the pelvic region, the cadaver's legs are spread wide, the ankles tied with clothesline to a long wooden bar, and raised high. That arrangement affords ideal viewing of the genitals as they are explored, dissected, and removed.

Of course a doctor needs to know how genitals work. Of course that imperative requires overcoming reluctance, squeamishness, modesty. But without a counterbalancing discussion of the humanity that is also present in the body parts—a conversation for which there is no time—doesn't that necessity compel students to distance themselves, to see anatomy instead of a human, just as later in their careers they may see a disease rather than a person?

"You start really early on separating what's on the table from people walking around," Abby said. "It's a coping mechanism. You have to learn to disassociate the science and studies from all the emotional stuff."

It doesn't always work. Sometimes the body's person comes through. "I had a hard time with the hands and the feet," Abby recalled. "And the nose. The nose. Not because I was grossed out, but because it was too human. I thought, 'I cannot do the nose.' I got the real sense of humanness for the body.

"I had to take a break. You just pass the scalpel and take a look outside for a while."

The other problem was that out in the real world, away from the lab, people started turning into anatomies on the hoof.

"I was walking up the stairs behind this girl in a halter top, and you could see all of these muscle groups. I thought, 'Whoa, this is weird. Is this what the rest of my life is going to be like?' Yes, and that's why you're taking this class."

Abby established a routine after each lab: a long shower, to remove the formaldehyde smell and to rinse away the emotions of the cutting. "Even if it was midnight, I didn't want that smell on my pillow, or its associations."

One other connection took place that semester, Abby said. "You realize, in cutting into human muscle, that we are just like other animals. Our muscle looks exactly like the muscle that you see nicely packaged in the supermarket."

In other words, meat. Students become so focused on what they must learn that the former human being under their hands becomes just so much London broil. This association arises so frequently each fall, thanks to anatomy educators all across the country, it is now virtually a medical-school cliché for first-year students to become vegetarians.

CHAPTER TWELVE

"TAKE FIVE YEARS"

Here is the fundamental problem in the quality of end-of-life care in America: The people we rely on to provide this help do not know how to do it. From the outset of their education to its conclusion, as much as a decade and $150,000 later, they are not being taught about death and dying. At virtually every level—clinical, practical, spiritual—they are unprepared. Excepting those rare individuals who through hard experience or uncommon openheartedness find themselves ready to face mortality, the breadth of physicians' ignorance about something they and all their patients will face is comprehensive.

It starts with their textbooks. In many academic disciplines, these books are only vaguely indicative of the accepted thinking on a given topic. History texts often disagree; literary anthologies routinely offer differing views of the canon. Not so in medicine.

"Textbooks serve as the cornerstone in the training of medical students and residents," Michael Rabow, M.D., writes in the *Journal of the American Medical Association*. What's more, he holds, the books serve as "authoritative references and reviews for more experienced clinicians, and as an important feature of professional orthodoxy and culture. Textbooks are central to clinical medicine, not only describing the expected best practices but also codifying the principles and standards of clinical care."

Textbooks, in other words, are the Bibles of behavior for students and seasoned practitioners alike. Thus, it was noteworthy a few years ago when researchers began scouring medical textbooks for references to end-of-life care. The results are alarming.

The first study, performed in 1999 by Annette Carron, D.O., reviewed four general textbooks, each a classic on internal medicine.

"Helpful information was rare," she writes. Any end-of-life discussion was limited to medical treatments, rather than making patients or families comfortable. Frequently in the books' world, patients' lives simply did not end. "Frankness about death was strikingly absent."

Perhaps it is understandable that the texts did not address such concerns as helping families cope, assisting patients who want to reconcile problem relationships, reckoning with the back-breaking cost of terminal care, or enabling people to attain spiritual calm. After all, these issues are largely nonscientific. But there is no justification for neglecting predictable medical dilemmas such as when to stop a kidney patient's dialysis, whether to use a feeding tube for an Alzheimer's patient who refuses to eat, or how long a person with failing lungs should be sustained by a ventilator.

A few books' shortfalls were so severe they verged on the comic. "Sometimes dead persons were termed 'non-survivors,'" Carron writes. The missing specifics added up to a larger implication, too.

"The fact that the medical profession and its classic information sources could so completely disregard the experience of dying and the opportunities to serve dying persons is perplexing," Carron says. "We need the information, practices and care systems that will improve outcomes for patients and families."

Carron did find one textbook worthy of praise, saying it "demonstrates a more straightforward honesty about the fact of death." The text she lauds is William Osler's *Principles and Practice of Medicine*. Osler, founder of the first U.S. medical school at Johns Hopkins University, published that book in 1899.

Today by contrast, "physicians cannot turn to general medical textbooks for guidance about advanced care planning, decision making, the effect of death and dying on the patient's family, or symptom management," Carron writes. Her advice, on the whole, was that "physicians should seek guidance from other sources."

The bad news is that those other sources turn out to be no better. Dr. Rabow led a team of University of California researchers in a study of fifty books used to train medical specialists. These texts address geriatrics, AIDS, infectious diseases, and other illnesses that regularly culminate in death. "Most disease-oriented chapters had no or minimal end-of-life care content," he says. "Specialty textbooks about certain diseases often did not contain helpful information on helping patients dying from those diseases."

Rabow's team took several approaches to their review, ostensibly to present the books in the most favorable light possible. But none was flattering. The most telling analysis was a simple count of the pages, to determine how many times end-of-life care issues were mentioned, regardless of the depth of discussion. Out of 34,845 textbook pages, 697 contained any reference whatsoever to end-of-life care. That's 2 percent.

"Chapters focused on end-of-life care were uncommon in some specialties (such as oncology, pediatrics and psychiatry) and were completely absent in the cardiology, infectious diseases, AIDS, neurology, pulmonary and surgery texts," Rabow writes.

The books were equally deficient in the nonmedical aspects of dying. "Consistently, there was a paucity of attention to the domains of spiritual, family and ethical issues at the end of life, and to the domain of physician responsibilities after death."

Rabow's use of the word *paucity* is apt, implying an impoverishment of imagination not only among the books' authors and editors but also on the part of a medical system whose reflexes emphasize intervention in diseases rather than care for people. Can you imagine an AIDS textbook that does not have a single chapter about dying? Or a book on geriatrics that barely mentions end-of-life care?

The situation is equally dire in nursing training. Betty Ferrell, Ph.D., performed an analysis of fifty nursing textbooks. Of 45,683 total pages, 902 address any end-of-life care topic—a rate of 2 percent. Of the books' 1,750 chapters, 24 are about the end of life—a 1.4 percent score.

A 1999 editorial in the *Journal of Palliative Medicine* renders a verdict on this state of affairs. Titled "A Failing Grade for End-of-Life Content in Textbooks," the opinion piece rightly notes that "nurses and physicians cannot do what they do not know. Inadequate knowledge is a key barrier to good care at the end of life, and inadequacies in textbooks are at least partly to blame."

Of course, textbooks are one small facet of the training that college graduates receive in their four-year pursuit of an M.D. Lectures, labs, and other course content are larger factors, obviously, and students' introduction to clinical work with actual patients can be profoundly formative.

Yet these areas also remain demonstrably weak. From the mid-1980s onward, article after article—in such publications as the *Journal of the AMA*, the *Archives of Internal Medicine*, the *Journal of Cancer Educa-*

tion, Medical Education—has concluded that medical students' exposure to the physical and emotional needs of people at the end of their lives is insufficient.

The problem is one of "failing to educate health professionals about how to provide superior, or even competent, care for dying patients," the Institute of Medicine has declared. The institute's 2001 book *Approaching Death* is widely considered the definitive study of the quality of end-of-life care in America. It is a damning treatise.

"Many physicians can recount how poorly prepared they were as students and residents to encounter dying patients and their families," the institute's report continues. "Deficiencies in undergraduate, graduate, and continuing education reflect a medical culture that defines death as failure and ignores care for dying people as a source of professional accomplishment and personal meaning."

The evidence of that culture is obvious. In 1996 only six of the nation's 126 medical schools required students to take courses on end-of-life care. In a survey of third-year medical students, "41 percent had never heard a physician talking with a dying patient, 35 percent had never discussed care for dying patients with an attending physician, and the great majority had never been present when a surgeon told a family that a patient had died," the institute reports. "Almost half the students could not remember *any* consideration of death and dying in the curriculum."

Medical students themselves are increasingly aware of the shortcoming in their training. Heather Fraser, M.D., of the School of Medicine at the University of Colorado Health Sciences Center, surveyed fourth-year medical students at six schools around the country.

About half the students said they felt "prepared" for providing end-of-life care. But when it came to details, such as whether students felt ready to manage actual symptoms, discuss end-of-life issues with patients, or understand the cultural and spiritual aspects of terminal care, the preparedness scores fell to as low as 21.9 percent. "Many students did not have exposure to end-of-life experiences at all," Fraser writes.

William Nelson, Ph.D., of the New York City–based National Center for Ethics, summarizes the situation plainly: "Graduating medical students are inadequately trained in the care of the dying."

The center is part of VHA, an alliance of 2,400 nonprofit health-care organizations, and Nelson was speaking on behalf of Choice in Dying, a five-year effort to expand public awareness of end-of-life care options. The group, which included nationally recognized figures in medicine, law, theology, and ethics, reported its findings at the 1999 meeting of the American Association of Cancer Educators:

> *Although most medical school curricula include some material about death and dying, most of this content is offered as an elective or as part of a much broader required course. . . . The result is a fragmented approach that one observer suggests represents a well-established pattern of neglect of medical education in the care of the dying. Clearly, a greater commitment to teaching end-of-life issues in medical schools is needed, along with improved organization, faculty development and planned integration of content into existing or new programs.*

Nelson's point about faculty development is meaningful for a basic reason. Today's medical-school professors, in general, were trained in a time of different sensibilities. Doctors routinely withheld bad news from patients; medicine had all the answers. Death was failure. Today these professors cannot teach what they do not know.

The Association of American Medical Colleges defends the status quo. AAMC publications say that "teaching about death and dying is available as part of an existing course at 112 medical schools (96.1 percent). Over two thirds (67.8 percent) of 1998 U.S. medical school graduates believe that they had received an appropriate level of training in death and dying."

It's not enough. The medical schools' efforts represent progress, perhaps, but the AAMC has overlooked the outcome. National polls show that people consistently and overwhelmingly criticize the quality of their loved ones' end-of-life care. Experts share the public's view, too. The Institute of Medicine has concluded that "dying is too important a part of life to be left to one or two required lectures, or to be set aside on the grounds that medical educators are already swamped with competing demands for time and resources."

One of the more persuasive voices echoing that opinion is Dr. Ira Byock. Former president of the American Academy of Hospice and Palliative Medicine, Byock directed a $28 million Robert Wood Johnson Foundation program that scoured the country seeking the best practices in end-of-life care, and then spread those success stories. From the unlikely base of Missoula, Montana, Byock helped build a nationally recognized hospice program—not solely as an administrator but as a physician providing care to patients.

Byock has the mild affect you might expect of a man who has spent decades in the presence of people who are dying. He is soft-spoken, thoughtful when listening, quick to smile. But ask Byock his opinion of medical education on the care of the dying, and he slams both hands on his desk.

"It is inexcusable. I have been hearing medical school deans say for twenty years that they only have four years for medical school and so many subjects to cover, that there isn't enough time to teach people how to deal with death. I say, then take five years. Take five. Otherwise, we are teaching pilots to take off without teaching them how to land."

Byock says one reason medical students aren't taught how to deal with dying is that the instructors themselves are afraid of death. In addition, medical science is reluctant to admit that for every single patient eventually its methods and disciplines fail. So the educational emphasis goes elsewhere. The priorities are backward, Byock says.

"Today you cannot graduate from medical school without two hundred hours of obstetrics," he says. "Even though very few doctors will actually ever deliver a baby, and even though only fifty percent of the population will ever be at risk for an obstetric intervention, still three hundred hours is the standard.

"Yet death is something virtually every doctor will confront in his or her career, and one hundred percent of the population is at risk of needing effective end-of-life intervention. And death gets twenty-four hours in medical school. Only twenty-four. And at most schools, even that estimate is being generous."

CHAPTER THIRTEEN

A PIECE OF CAKE

W hat about after medical school? Do residency programs overcome the end-of-life-training deficiency?

A 2003 survey of residents at Montefiore Medical Center, part of the Albert Einstein College of Medicine in the Bronx, gives some indication. That study first faults the education residents received before their clinical rotations began: "Medical students currently provide care to few patients who die in hospital, and often graduate without ever witnessing a patient death."

That makes the residency experience all the more crucial, argues the study's author, Charles Schwartz, M.D.

The opportunities for training are vast, he writes. Residents in oncology and intensive-care rotations are working in "powerful locations" for learning palliative care. Likewise the growth in care delivered at patients' homes means residents can learn how to treat people outside the hospital setting. But the new doctors are benefiting from neither opportunity, Schwartz writes.

Residents amplified the point in their survey responses: 59 percent of them said faculty teaching of end-of-life care was "adequate" or worse.

Despite the educational potential of oncology and ICU rotations, Schwartz continues, "only 11 percent of residents rated oncology rotations as relevant to their end-of-life training, and only 18 percent rated ICU rotations as relevant."

Without faculty leadership, Schwartz says, residents failed to learn even so much as how to identify patients whose death was near. That left them far from knowing "how to deliver bad news, work with patients and families in treatment planning and provide these patients with optimal care."

Schwartz's study was limited, involving residents at a single hospital. Unfortunately, the deeper the research looks, the worse the results appear.

Patricia Mullan, Ph.D., of Michigan State University, researched end-of-life-care education in thirty-two internal-medicine residency programs. Her work set aside specialists, focusing instead on the generalist physicians who provide care in the majority of end-of-life situations. She didn't just test the residents, either; Mullan assessed their teachers' knowledge, too. In all, 1,410 residents and faculty took her thirty-six-question multiple-choice clinical test—which means that the correct answer was right there on the page. They also answered eighteen additional questions concerning such nonmedical issues as ethics and communication skills.

They failed the test. The median score was 57 percent.

"Poor scores in the knowledge examination among both residents and faculty reflected the lack of required training in pain and hospice care," Mullan concludes.

Insufficient instruction in controlling pain reveals a disconnect between doctors and patients that extends well beyond end-of-life care. After all, if a person falls on the stairs and hurts his ankle so badly that he goes to the emergency room, he is not immediately worried about whether it is a sprain or a strain or whether the injured tissue is a tendon or a ligament. What he cares about is that it hurts. Pain is usually patients' most urgent concern, though it is rarely doctors' primary focus.

The implications of that gap are most acute in end-of-life situations, when nonmedical needs are many, because people cannot attend to emotional or spiritual matters while their minds are clouded with pain. The physical torment must be under control first. Only then can doctors, families, and patients address the nonphysical issues.

Mullan found other faults as well: "Internal medicine residents have poor skills in conducting advance directive discussions and discussing resuscitation orders crucial to appropriate end-of-life care planning. Neither interns nor faculty were consistently accurate in assessing treatment preferences. Resident and faculty knowledge of ethical principles is poor, and many barriers exist to effective ethics teaching."

How did this happen? When Mullan asked residency-program directors about obstacles to better end-of-life-care training, 26 percent said that "faculty have poor skills in residency evaluation and feedback." Nine-

teen percent said that "there is little buy-in from residents about the need
to improve end-of-life care"; 41 percent said that "there is no or little time
for new curricular elements."

Mullan's conclusion sounds distressingly familiar: "Existing internal
medicine residency education lacks training for end-of-life care."

Even now, in other words, new doctors perpetuate the knowledge
deficit of their predecessors. Even now they do not know what the possibilities for a meaningful end of life may be. They do not know about the
incredible opportunity that they and their patients are missing.

IT WOULD BE ONE THING if the shortfall in medical education were only
technical, merely a matter of finding the right textbook or carving a few
more hours out of medical school to address the needs of the dying. Unfortunately, the problems are primarily ones of attitude.

"My first year as an intern, I had a patient admitted, a lovely lady, but
she was very uptight," recalled Colin Murray Parkes, M.D., in the documentary *Pioneers of Hospice*.

"She couldn't talk about her feelings about her illness," Parkes said.
"And I'd been trying to get through to her, because I knew she was like an
unexploded bomb. There were loads of things that wanted to come out.
But she was just too frightened of it.

"I was visiting the ward as she was opening a packet, and she said,
'Would you like a piece of cake, Doctor?' I thought this would be a great
opportunity to get close to her. I sat on the bed, chatting with her, with this
piece of cake in my mouth, sharing our feelings about what was happening.

"At that moment a senior doctor walked onto the ward, walked off
again. A moment later, a nurse appeared. She came up and said Dr. So-
and-so wants to speak to you.

"I was given a serious rap over the knuckles. I was told I must not get
close to patients. It was utterly unprofessional for me to sit on a patient's
bed, holding a piece of cake, and this was going to create big problems for
me because I would get too involved.

"This sort of message, of not getting involved, keep your distance, was
what we were being taught to do. I knew it was wrong. With that lady, I was
just breaking through. . . . It really highlighted for me the gap between the
dogma of what was being taught at the time and what was really needed."

The temptation to assign blame in a story like this is strong. But
quick condemnation of Dr. So-and-so overlooks the many positives of a

medical can-do mentality. It is part of the wonderfully charismatic medical culture to act, to treat illness, to intervene—ideally, in a dramatic or heroic way—rather than to accept. When the challenge at hand was sudden death, this attitude resulted in thousands of heart attacks prevented, strokes survived, accidents avoided, longer life spans—in all, a breathtaking success.

The same cultural bent cannot work, though, in an era of gradual dying. It cannot work, because eventually everyone dies. Doctors may yet be trained to believe the contrary, but there is no cure for mortality. Some of the sadder stories in medicine involve not ordinary patients who receive shoddy care, therefore, but physicians who discover these cold realities when they find themselves on the other end of the stethoscope.

Balfour Mount, M.D., founded the Palliative Care Service at the Royal Victoria Hospital in Montreal. A longtime professor at McGill University, he developed cancer and had surgery to remove a portion of his esophagus. Afterward a group of doctors on rounds came to his room.

"The one person who clearly was meant to report on my condition tentatively approached the bed, and got to about my knee, my right knee," Mount recounted in *Pioneers of Hospice*. "I was waiting for him to come up, say hello, and ask me how I was.

"And he didn't. In fact, he never looked at me. He looked at my right knee for a moment, and then turned to the entourage at the end of the bed, and said in rapid fire what my blood gases were and how I was in terms of vital signs. But what struck me was the total lack of connection between these four or five young surgeons and myself. There was no eye contact. There was no discussion. There was no 'Well, how are you, Dr. Mount, how are you feeling today? How did the night go?'

"My fantasy was that there was a wall between us, a plate-glass window that we all couldn't see but that was totally preventing our relating.

"And I was having that thought when the young doctor at this end turned to the young one beside her, and said, 'It's too bad, isn't it? Oh well. He should have five or six good months left.'

"And that was it. And then they turned and walked off."

THE NARROW CLINICAL MIND-SET is a problem not only for older adult patients. It is pervasive, as the story of Betty Ferrell, Ph.D., illustrates. Ferrell, based at the City of Hope Hospital in Los Angeles County, California, is one of the nation's preeminent pain experts. She led a successful initiative to improve pain management in California. She lectures around the country on improving palliative care. If anyone is equipped to make certain the job is done right, Ferrell is.

Then she delivered a son prematurely. Andrew was placed in a neonatal intensive-care unit.

"When the hope was that my son would survive, of course we wanted all measures possible," Ferrell said. "But when that was done, there was no discussion whatsoever, like 'Let's get the chaplain here' or 'Let's get to a private place.'

"The problem is that the NICU is like the emergency room or other critical care, and these systems are designed to save lives. The mentality is, 'What we do is save lives, prolong lives,' and you the family member are left standing there. Or we have doctors standing in hallways saying, 'What do you want to have done with your son?' This is the wrong place."

After three months Andrew reached his small life's final moments. "I found myself pleading with the NICU staff, arguing with them to please disconnect all the tubes so at least I can hold my son while he dies."

Such wrenching experiences are common, Ferrell said. "Today, right now, somebody is dying in an emergency room. And I can promise you that what is going to happen to them will not go well."

So many doctors and nurses have experienced problems that they formed an organization—Professionals with Personal Experience in Chronic Care—to tell their stories and advocate for improvement. The founder of PPECC was Robert Kane, M.D., of the University of Minnesota, a leading researcher in geriatrics and author of hundreds of publications during his long career.

In 1999 his mother had a stroke. "Our mother took great pride in her independence," Kane said. "She recovered an amazing amount of function after rehabilitation." The family assembled a program of women coming to help the eighty-four-year-old with household tasks for a few hours each day and to provide company at lunchtime. This approach worked for months, until Kane's mother had a series of problems related to her congestive heart failure and infections.

"Every time she went to the hospital, her condition deteriorated because she'd changed her environment, she was confused, she got agitated, they put her on psychoactive drugs. It was just a repeating cycle of events. They were . . . produced by the treatment."

Despite the fact that health care was making her sicker, and despite his long experience caring for elders, Kane could not obtain appropriate treatment for his mother. "I was livid. I could spit nails. I knew what needed to be done."

Finally the family placed her in an assisted-living facility with special programs for people with dementia. Kane knew the owners personally. His mother "spent nine months there, hating being among 'crazy people.'" Then she moved to a nursing home, where she died three months later.

"Thirty years of practice and research wasn't worth a damn," Kane said. "Knowing people, being able to have direct contact, being able to seek out the best and the brightest in the field, didn't make the system work."

That is not good news for the common man. "If somebody with my experience and my knowledge couldn't make the system work," Dr. Kane said, "what chance does the ordinary person have?"

Kane put ads in medical journals asking if other clinicians had experienced similar frustrations. He received more than two hundred responses, some of which are collected on the PPECC Web site.

From Kansas to Minnesota, doctors describe what they call "medical mismanagement" that caused needless emotional and physical suffering. PPECC aims to build not only on these stories, but also on the credentials of the people telling them, to raise awareness of problems with chronic-illness care. The organization's mere existence proves a further point: Even among practitioners there is a growing understanding that medicine is not designed for the kind of care people need today at the end of their lives.

How bad is doctors' lack of understanding about those patients' needs? One indicator is what passes for professional development—that is, instructional articles in medical journals.

Timothy Quill, M.D., a recognized expert in end-of-life-care issues, unwittingly revealed the depth of doctors' shortcoming in a journal article about how to give a person bad news. It's not that Quill gave wrong advice; it's just that his counsel was so obvious that doctors ought not to need it.

"It is incumbent on the physician to ensure that the information about the diagnosis is accurate," Quill advises. "Bad news should be delivered in a face-to-face encounter. It is not a task to be delegated or to be done in an indirect way, such as over the phone. Exploring, tolerating and listening to a patient's response to bad news are perhaps the most vital steps."

Quill, with a hospice nurse as coauthor, cannot be faulted for suggesting that doctors listen closely to distraught patients. He is quite correct. But the mere fact that this notion must be explicitly stated is troubling. What Quill carefully articulates to his physician-reader is information that patients and their families would consider so basic as to not even require saying, much less being published in a medical journal. Do doctors truly not know that they should make absolutely sure a person has cancer before they say so? Are physicians actually unaware that they should not deliver negative test results over the phone?

CHAPTER FOURTEEN

"*THIS* WAS MEDICINE"

I will never forget," said Zail Berry, M.D., "two completely different patients, two completely different responses from the medical community."

One case taught her about what the clinical world values most. Another taught her about what patients value most. Together, they educated Berry about the vast chasm between the two.

It was 1988. Berry was a third-year internal-medicine resident in San Francisco when a man came into the emergency room with a severely diseased heart and a pulse of about 30. "The blood pressure was low, he was completely out of it." Dr. Berry, in the coronary-care unit, was paged to admit the patient to the hospital.

The ER doctor was trying to "pace" the patient's heart—that is, use a pacemaker wire to establish a life-sustaining heart rhythm, but on an emergency basis rather than in surgery. The technique uses a vein in the neck as a pathway to the heart. The doctor watches a monitor that follows the wire's progress. Once the wire hits the heart muscle, the physician turns on the pacemaker. The electric impulse dictates the heart rate, literally a lifesaving move.

"That's what the ER doc was trying to do," Berry recalled. "But she couldn't get capture, couldn't get the wire to conduct electricity to the man's heart muscle. There was a lot of concern. This guy was not getting a whole lot of blood to his brain."

The ER doctor asked Berry to try pacing the heart "transthoracically." That approach uses an eight-inch needle, inserted under the ribs and aimed for the heart, to attach the pacemaker wire. Instantly, she focused her concentration.

"It happens very fast, you don't have much time," she said. "The rest of the world goes away and you're right there."

After a few seconds "I got capture, sewed it in place, and hoped it didn't move. It was pretty dramatic."

So was the response from her peers and mentors. Some praised her for her skill. Others teased her for planning to be a general practitioner. "The next day the whole hospital was talking about it. 'Hey, Berry, what are you doing in primary care?' and this whole macho bullshit thing."

The man was hospitalized for a month. His care required frequent painful procedures and time on a ventilator. Finally he went home.

"He came back to the ER in a couple of weeks, dead on arrival," Berry said. "I'd basically tortured the guy for a month. And for what?"

It's not that she is anti-intervention, she said. "Heck, what's a few pokes if you can be made good as new? When he died, though, I felt terrible for all we put him through. Flogging a dead horse."

The man's case was especially poignant because it came at roughly the same time as Grace. She was a thirty-eight-year-old San Francisco bohemian, an organic food eater and crystal wearer, with a large extended family and a case of heartburn that wasn't responding to medication. Eventually doctors found stomach cancer.

"There's not a lot you can do," Berry said. "It's a very bad, nasty cancer. I helped break the news to her family."

Grace was scheduled for chemotherapy. "Those were the days when people stayed overnight, but she didn't want to, she had really not wanted to be in the hospital." She had a permanent catheter inserted, and Berry agreed to make house calls so Grace could receive the chemo as an outpatient. After several rounds of treatment, Grace stopped. Then she called Berry.

She "felt like she should have a doctor," Berry said. "I said, 'What happened to your oncologist?' She said, 'He told me to come back when I wanted more chemo.'"

Berry spares few obscenities to describe that oncologist when she tells the story. But she has only positive words for the experience that followed. She discovered new possibilities in her profession. She learned about a dying person's remarkable powers. Most important, she experienced a doctor-patient relationship beyond any she'd known before.

"Grace was an amazingly calm, serene, peaceful person," Berry said. "You just wanted to be around her."

She began gaining water weight in her belly, a common symptom with that particular cancer. "She looked like a pregnant twenty-five-year-old woman. People would say, 'When are you due?' She would give a calm, reassuring smile. 'Oh no, I'm not pregnant. You see, I have cancer.'"

Berry made more house calls. Whenever she arrived the family had food ready. Once a sibling's girlfriend asked, "When she dies, is it going to be gross or anything?" Berry used the question as an opportunity to explain the different ways people typically succumb to cancer.

Eventually Grace's family called to say she had changed and was not doing well. "I was leaving that weekend to go skiing. The family was panicked. I told them who I had arranged to cover for me while I was away. Then I went upstairs and examined her. Grace didn't respond.

"When I told her I would be going out of town, she opened her eyes—not a judgment, just getting it. . . . She died the next afternoon, before I left. I've always felt it was like a favor to me. It was the first time I had seen someone control the timing of their death."

Berry went on the trip. "I was fairly bummed out. So I went to the house after and saw pictures, saw the container her ashes were in."

The contrast between Grace and the paced man was powerful for a doctor in the middle of her training, Berry said. "I was elevated in the eyes of people for pacing that guy, and what good did I do that man? I tortured him. And after Grace died, I was supposed to feel like I had failed. But I felt good. I had helped her reach her goal of living with cancer without spending a night in the hospital.

"In fact, I felt that lots of people needed something I wasn't being trained to do. In fact, I felt like my profession was pretty badly screwed up."

Berry went and found the training she needed. For years she was medical director of an inpatient hospice center in Washington, D.C. Today she estimates she has attended more than three thousand deaths, and has devoted her career to helping people achieve good ones.

Along the way she also learned to advocate for herself. "My lawyer said my living will is the most exactly stated she's ever seen." She laughed. "And my husband knows I will haunt him into eternity if he keeps me alive against my instructions."

Meanwhile, strangers come up to Berry in the grocery store and give her a hug. "They say I helped their mother five years ago, something like that. There have been so many over the years, I can't possibly remember all the families. But these people remember me, and with incredible intensity."

Her decades of helping dying people has formed her in other ways, too. "The work has definitely made me more spiritual."

Berry's discovery seems less surprising in light of several studies of medical students who were exposed even briefly to end-of-life care. Their responsiveness is encouraging for them as doctors and for what it says about human nature. Researchers found that giving doctors-to-be a taste of hospice and palliative medicine not only increases their interest in caring for people at the end of their lives but also shapes their attitudes toward all patients.

In 1995 Northwestern University gave forty-four first-year medical students a quick hospice experience. The students were only a few months out of college, deep in the textbook phase of their education. But they spent an afternoon making home visits with a hospice nurse, then tagged along with the hospice's medical director for an afternoon.

Students later wrote about the experience. Many reported being anxious beforehand, uncomfortable during visits, and sad afterward. Many said they felt inadequate and intrusive. Spending time with dying people was intense and draining, the students said. All these emotions mirror what ordinary people experience when they are unfamiliar with death and find themselves in the presence of a person who is dying.

But witnessing hospice had uplifting effects, too. One student wrote that the doctor he followed "offered his hand to the patient, which he eagerly grasped and held during the entire interview, showing the effectiveness of contact for the physician to evoke trust and offer support to the ailing patient."

Another student wrote, "Her headaches seemed insignificant in relation to everything else going on in her life. But it wasn't. Her comfort was of immediate and significant importance, especially to the doctor."

Students said they appreciated the level of collaboration between doctors and nurses in hospice care, and the contributions of nurses in general. Hospice was markedly different from their hospital experiences because of what one student called "the emotional side." They wrote of learning that "the very purpose of palliative care is to deal with death in the most comfortable and caring way possible."

The students found that many dying people were not scary and in fact made efforts to put the doctors-to-be at ease. They discovered that "each patient is different and should be treated accordingly. Patients, no matter what their condition, are people and deserve just as much respect."

These reactions "may merely reflect on how desperately a lecture-hall-bound student yearns for 'real life,'" writes Drs. Kathy Johnson Neely and Douglas Reifler. "But it may also reflect on the genuine compassion and empathy inherent in our students. Most certainly, it encourages us in medical education to nurture this through the long and grueling years of medical education."

And beyond. Many of the doctors-to-be wrote that they would prefer hospice care at the end of their own lives and that their exposure to it would influence their career choices.

"As we drove back to my medical-school-three-block-world," one student wrote, "I hoped that I'd do home visits as a doctor. Medicine in the hospital or doctor's office seems so limited compared with this."

The students provide quite a contrast to Dr. Berry's "macho" medical world. All this from just two afternoons out of four years of medical school.

An even stronger story comes from Thomas Jefferson University in Philadelphia. A survey there involved third-year students. By that time the students have completed much of the classroom work and have begun clinical rotations. Many of the university's third-year rotations include six weeks of family medicine, with one week spent in the community. One year, students attended a single class on hospice and palliative care before spending a day accompanying a hospice nurse on home visits. Then the students were required to write "reflection papers."

Again the students' attitudes beforehand reflected normal anxiety, due to unfamiliarity with death. But writing about what they had learned afterward, they revealed the enormous potential in caring for people who are dying. The students' insightfulness merits quoting at some length.

- On where dying should occur: "It made sense that this man chose to die in his own home, surrounded by loved ones, in a familiar atmosphere, while being made comfortable by the hospice doctors and nurses. The other alternative is to stay in the hospital and be traumatized in attempts to avoid the unavoidable."

- On empathy: "For three years now I have been trying to come to terms with the notion of the sacred, esteemed, professional 'doctor-patient relationship.' Somehow I had gotten the idea that this relationship should be devoid of emotions. It took a woman like Nurse P. and a patient like Mr. J. to help me realize that it might actually be OK, normal and human to cry and to express emotions about a wonderful dying patient."

- On seeing the person rather than the illness: "I looked around their tiny living room, barely big enough to house the hospital bed they now had, at the photographs of the couple much younger, much healthier, arm in arm, all smiles. I was struck by a realization of how skewing the office walls can be, and how much of the individual they strip at the door. I imagined my feelings toward Mrs. P. if she were waiting for me in the office or hospital bed to visit. She would likely be distressed at being separated from her husband, depressed at being alone in the hospital, and agitated that she could get no one to take her outside for a cigarette. My feeling for this patient, and my empathy for her situation, and possibly even my attention to her complaints, would be drastically different." Another student further noted that "the frustration and anger that I was accustomed to seeing in the hospital were not present in the family members or the spouses" treated at home. Still another wrote that seeing patients in their homes "affords health care providers [an opportunity] to really understand who their patient is and what this patient's connection to the world is."

- On why meaningful dying matters: "My views on hospice and death have now transitioned. Instead of viewing hospice as a miserable existence for people who have no hope, my thoughts are that it is a peaceful way to live during the twilight of existence, and reflect on life, without all the distractions and frightening things at a hospital."

- On the role of families: "We helped to turn and clean him—a job that taxed both of us, since he was a tall man and dead weight. His wife had been doing this herself, four times a day, for several weeks." Another student added that "physicians need to remember that when they are taking care of a dying patient, they are actually taking care of everyone else in the household."

- On the physician's job: "You can only fail a patient if you fail to understand and respond to their needs. We may not be able to cure all of our patients, but if we can make them comfortable in the last moments of their lives, we will not have failed them."

- On the difference between dying and death: "Although patients in hospice care might be nearing the end of life, they value and enjoy every minute of their lives the way anyone else does."

Finally, one student wrote that through the human dimensions of hospice, "I came to understand that *this* was medicine, and this was so much greater than my naive ideas of complete cures and miraculous recoveries, which are joyous events when they occur but unfortunately are too few and far between; that the true practice of medicine is not the miraculous cure of a disease but the total care of a person."

If the third-year students gained this much wisdom from one class and one day, there is great hope yet for the medical profession. Their eloquence proves that they understood. Dying with dignity became concrete, something they saw with their own eyes.

A SIMILAR AWAKENING occurred for a group of twenty-seven new interns whom James Hallenbeck, M.D., of Palo Alto followed through a four-week hospice rotation. These were people two years further along in their medical training than the students at Thomas Jefferson; they were now M.D.s.

Yet most of the interns had no experience in caring for people who were dying, and only two had the knowledge that comes from losing close relatives. A questionnaire beforehand revealed that the interns did not think they would learn much from the rotation, did not think medical care would be "burdensome" to patients, and overwhelmingly thought that nursing-home and hospice work would be professionally "undesirable."

Four weeks later they were a different group of doctors.

"I believe I will be more conscious about aggressiveness of care in the terminal stages of life, consulting with competent patients, family members," one resident wrote.

The interns also said they learned "the importance of understanding where a patient is in relation to death, and being open and honest with patient and family so that death can occur in a way that the family and the dying patient can feel good about and come to terms with—if possible."

More broadly still, one wrote that "the issues and concepts concerning patient comfort can be applied to all my patients, not just the terminally ill."

The young doctors reported being better equipped to deal with their own loved ones' death. They said they were glad to have been exposed to hospice before advancing to their specialized training. Offered an opportunity to give criticism of the program, they had none.

Care of the dying humbled these interns at the same time it taught them. Their comments reveal that far from objecting, they loved it: "I think it was great to have a break from the technical detailed responsibilities of internship, and have more opportunity to think/focus on the dying process from a spiritual/emotional side."

CHAPTER FIFTEEN

"MAYBE I CAN MAKE YOU LAUGH"

Medical students and residents are only a subset of the health-care world, of course. They are earlier in their careers, and thus more likely to accept new notions of care and new attitudes toward patients. The greater unknown is how responsive seasoned practitioners might be if they were exposed to hospice and palliative care. So far there is not a wealth of data on the topic. But there are a few promising signs.

For example, there is the one-week intensive in hospice and palliative care run jointly by the Robert H. Lurie Comprehensive Cancer Center and Northwestern University medical school's Division of Hematology/Oncology. First, professional caregivers complete a twenty-five-question examination of their knowledge of medical issues for terminal patients. Their performance on that exam directs the education they receive during the week. Thus, the class is customized to their deficits. But, appropriately, the program is not all factual. Doctors' interviews with patients are videotaped, too, in order to reveal their strengths and weaknesses in communication skills.

Most people enrolled in the early sessions already had some interest or experience in end-of-life care, writes Charles von Gunten, M.D., in a report on the program. Unlike other palliative-care courses, which "have not been effective in changing cancer pain management," he notes, the Northwestern approach makes a difference. Attendees were surveyed about their views on the program six months later, using a 1–5 scale (with 5 being best). In response to the statement "the experience was worth the time and effort," the average score was 5.0. For "I would recommend this experience to others," again it was 5.0. The average response to "my current efforts are helping to change the way dying patients and their families are cared for in the broader environment in which I work" was 4.9. When participants were asked what the best part of the experience was, von Gunten says, "all wrote copious comments."

It is tempting to overstate the significance of the scores. After all, the program involves only one week out of an entire medical career. By contrast, palliative-care specialists in the United Kingdom must complete a four-year residency and a fellowship. And 100 percent of Canadian medical schools require students to study palliative care. Nevertheless, U.S. doctors' response to the Northwestern program suggests that the basics of end-of-life treatment can be learned in short order and that people who undertake this training are universally glad they did.

It won't be easy to make these small gains widespread. "Because this area has been neglected in medical education," von Gunten writes, "a substantial number of people who are already in practice need additional training. Approximating traditional residency or fellowship training for the thousands of physicians and other health care providers in practice who need additional education in this area is not practical."

Yet Northwestern is attempting to do just that with EPEC, a physician program originally offered by the American Medical Association. Education on Palliative and End-of-life Care is a two-and-a-half-day immersion for nurses, technicians, clinical ethicists, and, above all, doctors.

The hundred or so EPEC students in each session pay nine hundred dollars for lectures on gaps in the care of people toward the end of their lives, and on legal issues such as how to withhold or withdraw care properly. They learn the principles of palliative care: that patients should plan the treatment they receive, should write advance directives to guide that care, and should have their pain managed properly. The idea is never to hasten death but to provide choices so that people can maximize the quality of their remaining life.

The meat of EPEC comes later in the program, in smaller group classes. Michael Preodor, M.D., a Northwestern medical-school professor who is the director of EPEC, stressed the importance of the small-group dynamics.

"We have to apply what we know about how physicians learn, and how adults in general learn," he said. "Usually information is conveyed in grand rounds lectures. But what doctors take away from a didactic presentation before an audience of hundreds is very little. Their behavior doesn't change. The difference-maker in EPEC is the small groups, with interaction, role-playing, nitty-gritty real-world predicaments."

The group sessions concern such topics as communicating bad news, controlling patients' pain, treating depression and other psychological problems, managing symptoms like nausea or difficulty in breathing, and providing special care during a person's last hours.

Each session begins with a "trigger tape," Preodor said, which brings up many of the issues doctors hesitate to raise, much less discuss.

"When a patient brings up the idea of a physician-assisted suicide," Preodor gave as an example, "the request usually is based on issues of suffering. The patient is in pain, or some degree of disability, or more commonly feels like a burden on others. Now, we oppose assisted suicide, and it is illegal everywhere but Oregon. But that does not make the patient go away. Doctors learn that by addressing suffering, by finding out the cause and treating it, these requests nearly always go away."

Programs like EPEC contribute to progress in patient care, albeit slowly, Preodor said. "I remember twenty-six years ago when I first began this work, I felt like I was very isolated. I would fight with pharmacies to make a morphine elixir so I could manage patients' pain. I broke my neck trying to get people to do this. Since then, the drug companies decided that they could make a profit by making a long-acting morphine. So then there were fifteen hundred drug reps in doctors' offices, talking about pain management. There is progress. I'd like it to be faster, but we're doing okay."

What is the effect of exposing doctors to the solemn but rich rewards of caring for people at the end of their lives? It varies. Some find the work so compelling that they choose to specialize in palliative medicine. Others pursue medical specialties as planned, but informed by a new sensitivity to patient comfort. Still others take dramatic turns in their careers.

Doctors like Berry, who learned from Grace and the man whose heart she paced, fit into the first category. The other two reactions better describe a physician like Terry Rabinowitz, M.D.

Rabinowitz was a fully trained dentist completing a pediatric gum disease fellowship in Ohio when he was asked to treat an elderly man with mouth sores. It turned out that the man had cancer. Rabinowitz had never seen the disease up close before. The patient's illness was advanced, but he felt much more comfortable when his mouth sores lessened. The two men conversed long after each day's treatment was finished. Then one day Rabinowitz arrived to find the patient's room empty.

"It had never even occurred to me that he would die. That's how ignorant I was. I wasn't dealing with life and death, I was taking care of kids and their teeth. Well, I sat on his bed and I cried. I can't say why. I guess I liked him. As I thought about it, I realized I had made a little difference for him. And once I'd had that feeling, I couldn't stop thinking about it."

Rabinowitz quit dentistry and went to medical school, even though that meant another seven years of school and training.

"I knew the whole time what field I wanted to pursue." He became a consulting psychiatrist, specializing in the needs of terminal patients. "I look at the end of life as a pyramid. The top is death. Everything below that is treatable."

Dr. Rabinowitz typically meets patients in intensive care or some other waiting room to eternity. He helps them determine their final priorities, face demons, and prepare themselves. Sometimes patients want to heal old rifts, and he readily serves as mediator. But Rabinowitz is no Pollyanna: Sometimes people actually want permission to let old animosities remain.

"One great old guy just really didn't want his ex-wife to come barging in and inflict herself on him at the end of his life. We arranged visitors' orders for his room, on the door and on his chart, so only certain people were allowed in. He was so relieved, he was happy like a little kid. Think of that: Just by helping him to validate his true feelings and giving him the small and reasonable thing he wanted, I made it possible for him to feel better—even as he drew nearer to death."

Sometimes a doctor's simple presence reassures patients. "Someone who is dying, they start giving up stuff. They may project that you are giving up on them. You have to be very careful that they don't get that message. You say right out loud, 'I am going to be here.' The worst thing that can happen for someone who is dying is if there's nobody around."

Rabinowitz says he works hardest to help patients define themselves not by their disease but by the lives they led before they were ill. "With anyone who is dying, I'll say, 'How long have you been dying? The dying is really consuming you, it's filling you up. But what about the other fifty-four years?'

"You are a lot of other things besides being a cancer patient. You're a good father. You're a basketball player. You're dying, sure, yes. But you're also a person who bakes wonderful bread or has fallen arches or just visited the Washington Monument."

Reinforcing patients' individuality provides comfort, Rabinowitz says. And for himself, helping people achieve this perspective on their illness is a unique and enduring pleasure.

"From a psychiatric perspective, what we're trying to do is help whatever can be helped, to optimize the quality of life. A large part of that is to keep the level of dignity as high as it can be. We might see a person with metastatic cancer, for example. They're depressed, and refusing treatment that might prolong their life and enhance its quality. In that situation, there is work for us to do. There is suffering, and so there is a chance for us to help."

That work, which Rabinowitz admits is not for everyone, suits him well. "Maybe you go into a patient's room, and they have three or four tubes going into and out of them, and maybe it smells bad and they look like crap and they're going to die. But I became convinced that there was a chance to help the suffering of someone who was critically ill. I love the chance to help. I can't cure your illness, but maybe I can make you laugh."

MEDICAL LEADERS ARE just beginning to discover these possibilities. As the baby boomers among them experience the death of their parents, and of the first of their friends, they are starting to see their profession in a new and unflattering light. Some also see how dying has been transformed. They see the potential for a meaningful, high-quality life regardless of a person's medical circumstances.

Thus far, the result has been the birth of a few new facilities, as well as new teams within existing health-care institutions, geared toward improving the quality of care for people experiencing a slow fading of their lives. Dr. Byock launched a home-care and hospice program in Missoula, inspired in part by the death of his father. A young palliative-care program in Pittsburgh is growing steadily, adding doctors, nurse practitioners, researchers, and residents. At Mount Sinai Dr. Meier was a geriatrician with a focus on palliative medicine; now she runs an organization dedicated to spreading palliative principles and practices across the country.

A growing number of hospitals are also addressing nonmedical issues. Twenty years ago doctors relied on their own internal compasses to navigate decision making. Now many community hospitals have ethics committees, while larger medical centers have departments of clinical ethics. These doctors, nurses, theologians, and others have as their mission to guide families and patients through the difficult process of choosing how much care a person should receive at the end of his or her days. What is the situation, what are the options, what are the values that should guide this decision making? Families and patients learn the true prognosis, discuss the alternatives, and determine what suits them best.

The fundamental problem with these burgeoning programs is their isolation. The good places typically exist only because of a clinical leader who is personally committed to delivering competent end-of-life care. What America needs, as gradual dying becomes increasingly common, is systemic change. As Dr. Byock put it, travelers would not fly on an airline that had a few great pilots but the rest were a bit weak on landing. Likewise, the quality of care for people with terminal illnesses should not be a function of geography or luck.

Programs that teach doctors how to do the job right have the same drawback: They are too small and isolated. The Northwestern University intensive, success that it is, caters to fifteen physician-students at a time. Thomas Jefferson University's program of early exposure to hospice reaches only eighteen medical students a year. The Cleveland Clinic offered one of the nation's first postresidency fellowships in palliative medicine, starting in 1989. By the end of 2000, only ten doctors had completed the program.

Even the vaunted EPEC program, despite seven years of operating within the AMA, reaches only a hundred medical professionals at a time. With two sessions a year, EPEC can boast eighteen hundred graduates in its history. There are more than one million doctors in the United States.

The impact of these professional-development programs remains somewhat unclear.

"We are seeing a lot of advancement at an intellectual level," said Dr. Preodor, "but at a practical level we have a long way to go. The data shows that we can change doctors' attitudes, and we can change doctors' knowledge. We don't have evidence yet of whether we have changed doctors' behavior."

At this rate, how long before the islands of good care lose their isolation? How long until all Americans can depend on compassionate, personalized care at the end of their lives? Is that delay acceptable for the person who is suffering right now?

CHAPTER SIXTEEN

BARRIERS TO CHANGE

I n today's medical culture, even sincere and well-meaning practitioners remain ill-equipped to care for people who are dying. Yes, a shift is slowly beginning, and improvement is within reach.

There are obstacles, though, that have little to do with old attitudes or physicians' training. They are external to medicine, matters of policy, tradition, or law, and they present disincentives that will be difficult to overcome. These barriers are many; here, briefly, are five.

TO BEGIN WITH, medical education suffers from the weighty inertia common to the academic world. Remaking medical school and residency programs to accommodate gradual dying will not happen easily.

"Curriculum change is clearly a political as well as an intellectual process," holds the Institute of Medicine in its 1997 book, *Approaching Death*. "Departments have turf to protect, individual faculty have habits that are entrenched, and academic administrators bear scars from previous attempts at major changes."

The competition for resources, moreover, often comes from legitimate medical or social interests. "Improved care at the end of life can seem like just another in a continuing stream of claims for attention to such worthy issues as nutrition, aging, race and ethnicity, informed consent, substance abuse, environmental hazards and domestic violence," the institute's report explains.

Also not surprisingly, medical schools reward faculty whose research garners more money, whose scholarship wins greater recognition, and whose departments draw more students. Compared with genetic medicine, surgery, and other high-profile disciplines, end-of-life care is simply not sexy enough.

The immediate result is a climate of reluctance. The institute quotes a medical school dean who was being either pessimistic or realistic when he said, "Most deans would rather take a daily physical beating than try to make significant changes in the traditional curriculum."

The vast majority of doctors care about their patients and mean well. But when medical education continues to train physicians with an insufficient understanding of dying, they do not know how to treat patients in that most challenging, and potentially rewarding, phase of their lives.

A SECOND BARRIER to better care of the dying results from doctors' healthy skepticism about novel notions in medical care. This attitude stems not from ego but from caution. Physicians rarely embrace new tools, drugs, or procedures until those ideas have been published in a medical journal and have been subject to subsequent trial and debate. Widespread acceptance of generic prescription drugs, for example, took nearly twenty years.

Most doctors put even less stock in ideas based on criticism of the status quo. That reflexive reaction conflicts with progressive notions about end-of-life care, because too often the data to validate hospice methods do not exist.

"The quality of evidence on symptom management appears to be limited," the National Institutes of Health concluded in 2004, following a three-day State of the Science summit meeting.

That research shortcoming was one of many the NIH noted. When it comes to communicating with patients, "a majority of the studies have been done outside the United States, in small samples."

Likewise for spirituality, a crucial concern for people nearing the end of their lives, "research on interventions to improve spiritual well-being is very limited."

As for the role of families, "only a limited number of randomized clinical trials have been conducted with caregivers of patients near end of life. There is limited information aside from dementia and little information about culturally diverse populations."

Regarding the impact caring for the dying has on doctors and nurses, "there is a lack of data regarding which caregivers are at greatest risk for distress and which interventions are likely to relieve that distress."

The NIH even touched on the lack of knowledge about less traditional aspects of end-of-life care. For example, hospices often employ alternative-medicine ideas such as music therapy and healing touch. Data on the usefulness of such treatments, which many physicians find dubious to begin with, "suffer from [an] insufficient number of studies, small samples and weak study designs."

Some doctors confess privately to another, less scientific reason that they distrust palliative medicine and hospice: righteousness. Too many end-of-life care providers suffer from the malady of self-assigned superiority. No doubt their work is emotionally demanding, but the same can be said for many jobs in health care. Just as some surgeons reinforce the stereotype of an arrogant gunslinger, some people who care for the dying validate complaints that they behave as if they always know supremely better what ought to be done. Humility would go a long way toward winning friends among doctors who are not impressed by arrogance.

NO DISCUSSION OF CHANGES in health care is complete without considering financial issues. Eugenia Siegler, M.D., has documented this third obstacle to providing better end-of-life care: money. Siegler was a geriatrician at Brooklyn Hospital Center, where a palliative-care program thrived for several years—and then collapsed.

The need for the service was not in question. "None of the faculty, including myself, had formal palliative care training," Siegler says. "Staff failed to perceive patients' symptoms, emotions and spiritual needs, and residents in particular lacked communications skills necessary to provide palliative care."

The program began with an innovative idea: Instead of waiting for doctors to send patients to palliative care, nurses would screen patients for possible palliative referrals every day. Appropriate candidates would meet with an experienced nurse specialist unless the doctor specifically directed otherwise. Siegler "provided backup," she writes, "serving as physician authority to wheedle, cajole or otherwise convince reluctant house staff and attendings to shift their focus away from a strictly curative to a broader outlook that included palliative care."

The program enjoyed high volume—470 cases in the first eighteen months. Patients ranged in age from twenty-one to ninety-one. The program had appealing side effects, too. In addition to improving end-of-life care, the hospital developed better sensitivity to cultural diversity, no small matter in the melting-pot neighborhoods it served. There were bumps in the road—physicians were too glad to abdicate responsibility for palliative care to the new program rather than incorporate it into their practices, and pain management did not improve measurably. But the program's leaders spoke at national meetings, gave grand rounds talks at hospitals considering similar ventures, and otherwise showed every manifestation of success.

Then the grant funding the program's social worker dried up. Tight budgets throughout the hospital led the nurse expert to leave, too. Soon after, Siegler herself departed. Her parting shot: "The hospital lacks the capital to support not just a salary, but a program."

Isn't it odd that the kind of care virtually everyone will need at some point in their lives is somehow too expensive for hospitals to provide? Or, to put it more accurately, that hospice and palliative care do not generate enough revenue to be self-sustaining, compared with money-making services like orthopedic surgery?

Later chapters challenge this assumption, demonstrating how improving care of the dying could actually save money. Nevertheless, Siegler's experience proves that financial obstacles to change are formidable.

A FOURTH KIND OF CHALLENGE confronts doctors who, despite these disincentives, remain determined to care for people who are dying: criminal prosecutors.

Armed agents raided the Shasta County, California, clinic of general practitioner Frank Fisher, M.D., on February 18, 1999. He was charged with trafficking in drugs, defrauding the state health-insurance program of $2 million, and committing five murders. Prosecutors called Fisher a "drug dealing mass murderer." Unable to post a $15 million bond, Fisher spent five months in jail. The government seized his assets, and he faced a possible life sentence. Four patients' families filed wrongful-death suits against Fisher, alleging that their loved ones had died of pain-drug overdoses. Although the Medical Board of California did not revoke his license, a superior court judge placed sufficient conditions on Fisher that he stopped practicing medicine.

Fisher, a forty-five-year-old Harvard Medical School graduate, moved back in with his parents. Then he began a five-year legal ordeal to clear his name.

At a twenty-one-day preliminary hearing, details about the alleged murders emerged. One victim had died in a car accident. Another victim had not been a patient of Fisher's but received drugs stolen from one of his patients. A third victim was actually alive at the time of Fisher's arrest.

A judge threw out all the murder charges. Fisher still faced manslaughter charges, as well as twenty-six felony counts of Medi-Cal fraud. Then the manslaughter case evaporated, and the fraud case shrank to eight misdemeanor counts. Prosecutors maintained that Fisher had filed $4,300 in fraudulent claims to the state's health-insurance program, which had paid $1,125. Fisher's attorneys countered that the dispute, the result of confusion about Medi-Cal's complicated billing system, amounted to about $150. After a two-week trial, the doctor was found not guilty on all counts.

On February 2, 2005, just shy of the six-year anniversary of the raid on Fisher's clinic, the last of the wrongful-death suits was dismissed. Two of the four plaintiffs were ordered to pay Fisher damages.

"His ordeal lingers as a cautionary tale of what can happen to doctors who treat pain aggressively," wrote Sally Satel, M.D., adviser to the Substance Abuse and Mental Health Services Administration. "The red flags that rightly alert regulators to potential misconduct by doctors are, paradoxically, the very features that can also mark responsible care for intractable pain."

It's difficult for doctors. A small fraction of patients report pain only as a way to obtain drugs. Other patients develop a physical dependence on pain medication, cultivating a tolerance so that larger doses are required to control the same amount of pain. A small percentage—far less than media accounts might indicate—become addicted.

To prevent drugs from landing in the wrong hands, Texas mandated that doctors write prescriptions on a triplicate form. The outcome was different from the law's intent. Credible pain specialists, examining state records, determined that the share of drugs diverted from proper uses was only .08 percent. But the chilling side effect was that doctors prescribed pain control drugs in far lower amounts—54 percent less at one hospital alone. The trade-off for anticrime efforts, therefore, was patients' pain.

As the AMA's formal policy on pain management puts it, "Unbalanced and misleading media coverage on the abuse of opioid analgesics not only perpetuates misconceptions about pain management, it also compromises the access to adequate pain relief sought by over 75 million Americans living with pain."

These are serious issues for society to address. Police and prosecutors must reckon with the crimes committed by addicts seeking either drugs or money to buy drugs. Quite obviously, though, these concerns diminish if the patients are nearing the end of their lives. A bedridden cancer patient is not going to rob a convenience store to support his morphine habit. And what harm does physical dependence cause a person who will be alive only a few more weeks? Isn't the possible danger far outweighed by the potential for alleviating suffering?

There have been enough cases over the years of doctors abusing or dealing drugs that the answer is not to give all physicians free rein. Similarly, the small fraction of nurses who abuse drugs has hurt the whole profession. As with doctors, prosecutions of upstanding nurses from Maine to Minnesota to Montana reveal that the scale between pain management and law enforcement is tipped steeply toward preventing crime. Thus, it inclines away from comforting patients.

The practical issue is how the medical community and the law-enforcement community can come to an understanding so that physicians provide appropriate medicine to their patients and criminals go to jail.

In 2001 leaders on these issues began an effort to find the proper balance. Twenty-one health groups, from pain-management and palliative-care organizations to the American Medical Association, collaborated with the federal Drug Enforcement Administration. The result appeared in August 2004: "Prescription Pain Medications: Frequently Asked Questions and Answers for Health Care Professionals and Law Enforcement Personnel."

The Q&A received strong endorsements from pain specialists such as Russell Portenoy, M.D., chairman of palliative care at Beth Israel Medical Center in New York City. "We now have two serious societal problems— the undertreatment of pain, and drug abuse . . . that are intertwined through prescription pain medications. We address both problems in this document, and hope it will bring some clarity to the issue."

Instead, by October the document was no longer available. The DEA said it "contained misstatements" and "was not approved as an official statement of the agency."

It appears the antidrug worries prevailed. The AMA responded that "physicians who appropriately prescribe or administer controlled substances to relieve intractable pain should not be subject to the burdens of excessive regulatory scrutiny, inappropriate disciplinary action or criminal prosecution."

The collaborative effort was intended to reassure physicians; the DEA's hasty retreat had the opposite effect. A survey of thirteen hundred New York doctors found 60 percent concerned about being investigated for prescribing opiate-based drugs for noncancer pain, Dr. Satel said. A third said they frequently prescribe lower dosages than what is needed to control the pain.

It makes sense for doctors to protect themselves, their families, and their careers. Meanwhile, though, patients suffer.

John Nelson, M.D., president of the American Medical Association, drew this conclusion: "The most serious abuse of pain medication is its underuse."

THE FIFTH AND LARGEST obstacle to improved end-of-life care is one of attitude. Physicians' own apprehension about death and their professional emphasis on science combine to powerful effect.

That effect may be most evident among cancer doctors, according to Anthony Back, M.D., who practices in that specialty. "An oncologist who is uncomfortable with dying is more likely to offer another round of chemotherapy," he says. That pattern raises the question of whether his colleagues are "evil, or just oblivious."

Dr. Back answers his own query by citing the booklet *A Patient's Guide to Advanced Lung Cancer Treatment,* a consumer-education publication of the American Society of Clinical Oncology. There are, Back writes, chapters on "lung cancer histology, staging, chemotherapy, radiation, side effects and clinical trials. In the very last sentence of a chapter entitled 'After Treatment Ends,' readers learn that 'hospice for comfort care may be suggested.' That is as explicit as this booklet gets in describing death from advanced lung cancer."

It would be easy to dismiss the problem as insensitivity, but the reality is more complex. Oncologists do not specialize in cancer to help people die well, Back says, but to cure the disease. That is hardly a character flaw; millions of Americans are living today with cancers that were fatal a generation ago.

In that context of research and treatment success, overemphasis on science is perfectly understandable. Oddly enough, many patients place greater confidence in a surgeon whose manner is gruff and whose interpersonal skills are weak. Although there is no basis for this belief, somehow a rude or indifferent bedside manner implies if not greater prowess, then at least higher clinical priorities.

Caring for people at the end of their life requires a different set of skills. Attentiveness is more useful than attitude. Empathy counts more than ego. End-of-life care is less about science than about humanity, the human connections among patient and physician and family. Too many doctors today are not trained for that reality. It is inescapable, however; it looms in their future as practitioners, it awaits in their fate as mortals.

Here is a genuinely sad dimension of the health system's inattention to gradual dying: There is no recognition of the sorrow that doctors experience.

Think of it: They see death every day. Most have not been prepared to deal with it. They have no mechanism for experiencing the loss and eventually healing from it. Imagine the cumulative effect, over days and years and a career.

Because of the long-institutionalized combination of denying emotions and emphasizing a scientific approach to care, there is no system in place to reckon with physicians' own feelings. Whether they are medical students intimidated by a cadaver, or residents overwhelmed by the first death of a patient in their care, or seasoned physicians who believe in the value of their life's work yet now must witness the slow, cold truth about its limits, there is within the profession an enormous reservoir of grief. And the practitioners are not allowed to show it or talk about it. Like soldiers' stoicism about a past war, they carry the weight of their experiences with no means for unburdening themselves.

Robert Orr, M.D., knows the problem well. He had been a family doctor for eighteen years when a suffering patient asked him to help end her life.

"I can still remember her face," Orr said. "She was a mother of young children and had an advanced bone cancer, very painful, very."

Orr refused her request, saying that to aid in her dying would violate his Hippocratic oath. She asked him at least to increase her pain medication.

"I did not do that for her, either. The textbooks said that for a person of this weight, you only use so much morphine."

Orr followed the rules. "She suffered horribly. Her family watched her suffer, her husband, her children. I watched her suffer, too. But I did nothing. I behaved as I had been told. Finally she died. It was a relief to her family. But not to me. She has been with me ever since."

Her memory remained so strong, in fact, that Orr left family practice and began a second career in medical ethics. While most discussions about medical ethics are led by theologians, he said, there is an urgent need for these conversations to include physicians as well. Doctors certainly will not agree about every care decision, Orr conceded, but merely investing their time considering what is morally right will help them make wiser decisions—that is, ones determined less by flawed textbooks and governed more by the human need before them.

"I felt that I was well trained in medicine," Orr said, "but there was this big hole. It was a deficiency. I found a great reward in helping people with this. To relieve their pain and shortness of breath, to relieve anxiety, to help with spiritual concerns—it is almost as rewarding as saving a life, to make the end of life better."

After further training, Dr. Orr rose to become director of clinical ethics at the Loma Linda University Medical Center in California, and subsequently a consulting ethicist at hospitals in New York and New England. His task was to help families make informed choices for their dying loved ones—when to continue treatment, when doing so only prolongs suffering. He smiles easily, but his brow has a careworn look.

"I have realized that the textbooks were wrong. The right amount of pain medication, the only allowable definition of 'the right amount' if we are at all humane, is the dosage that alleviates pain. Anything less is irresponsible."

Orr worries that medical students follow those textbooks too closely. So he spends as much time educating doctors about options for end-of-life care as he does patients and families.

"There is a moral aspect to what we do, we doctors," he said. "And when we fail a patient as I failed that woman, it weighs heavily on our consciences." Orr took off his glasses and rubbed his forehead. "As well it should."

IF NOTHING ELSE, the increasing familiarity of some doctors with gradual dying can lead to discussions of those topics among their peers. An article in the *Journal of the American Medical Association*, for example, prompted a revealing letter to the editor from Bernard Siegel, M.D., of Woodbridge, Connecticut. The letter was titled "Crying in Stairwells: How Should We Grieve for Dying Patients."

"Again and again," Siegel writes, "physicians are crying in deserted corners of the hospital. Why is this happening? The answer is our lack of training, and the depersonalization that has become medicine. . . .

"Please, fellow physicians, don't cry in empty rooms, on stairwells or in locker rooms. Cry in public, and let the patients and staff heal you and see you are human. . . .

"As a surgeon, I had to come out from behind the cap, mask and gown and reveal a vulnerable human being. When that happened, I stopped being a fugitive and losing battles. I started helping people live, I found forgiveness, and I no longer had to ask, why me?

"I know physicians are human. We wear masks that prove it. But if we hide behind those masks, we are killing ourselves and the people we care for. Dealing with people, as opposed to caring for people, leads to depersonalization and pain for everyone. Help people live and don't be just a mechanic. Realize your patients are your resource, not your problem."

That letter sparked a reply from Stephen Schultz, M.D., of Rochester, New York. After describing how his training had prepared him somewhat to care for people who are dying, Schultz writes, "I am amazed that the emotional impact the patient might have on me was never discussed."

Then he recounts an incident from his days as an intern. "I diagnosed by ultrasound in the emergency department a late third-trimester fetal death. As I stared at the still heart, unable to believe what I was seeing, the attending physician walked into the cubicle. 'The baby's dead,' he announced in a flat monotone after glancing at the screen. He stood by the side of the bed, arms crossed, no hint of emotion, as the woman and her husband burst into tears. In that situation I wanted to stay, to share in their grief, but knew I could not do so without some display of my own sadness.

"I know that the sadness I felt originated both from my response to their loss and from my own grief as my wife and I struggled with infertility. But here the primary care provider stood, with a response entirely discordant with what I was feeling or wanted to do, and again I left the bedside to hide my grief."

Schultz goes on to say that despite his experiences, he does not share Siegel's view about doctors showing sadness in front of others. "The act of crying or other displays of grief are quite personal, and difficult for some to do at all, let alone in public. If the choice is crying alone or not at all, then by all means cry alone. We must first be comfortable with grief and its display within ourselves before we can share it."

About 2.5 million Americans die every year, 6,850 a day, with doctors present in the majority of cases. Considering how common a physician's experience of loss must therefore be, it is striking how little in the medical literature even mentions this unique sorrow. One report scratches the surface, though, and may inadvertently reveal a deeper issue.

The research took place at Massachusetts General Hospital, an eight-hundred-bed teaching hospital in Boston. The study surveyed clinicians about practical tasks they perform after a patient has died: verifying that death has occurred, preparing the body by removing tubes and equipment and by closing the mouth, cleaning the body and positioning it, notifying the family and providing consolation, discussing autopsy and organ donation, documenting the death, reviewing medical and personal reactions to the death among the clinical staff, and following up with the family—by attending a wake or funeral, sending a condolence note, providing autopsy results, or arranging bereavement care.

Grim functions all, they must be performed to some extent in every death. Clearly they will have some emotional effect on the person who performs them.

Clearly, too, there are better and worse ways that these tasks might be done. The survey found real problems. Only 15 percent of house staff removed lines or other tubes when a patient had died. Half never repositioned the body from its death posture. Imagine the trauma for families entering a room to find their deceased loved one in that condition.

One survey respondent "recalled another resident entering a room full of family members, determining that the patient was dead, and leaving the room without saying anything. The family was quite dissatisfied and complained to the clinical staff."

And likely never forgot the incident, either. But the anecdote reveals less a doctor callous about death than one incapable of dealing with it, and thus emotionally distanced to an inhumane degree.

Similar issues arose all through the survey. Only 30 percent of clinicians routinely raised the issue of organ donation. Only a third were ever involved in helping a family choose a funeral home or in elementary planning of other rituals. Half the residents surveyed did not regularly offer emotional support at the time of notifying a family of a death; 55 percent never provided a follow-up discussion or bereavement call, 77 percent had never written a note of condolence, and 88 percent never reviewed autopsy results with the family. Even less emotional tasks, such as filling out a death certificate, saw 80 percent error rates. Eighty percent.

This performance cannot be written off as ineptitude. Residents at Mass General are among the brightest and most competitive in the country. These young doctors are definitely skilled enough to perform the after-death tasks competently. There is another explanation.

"Several house staff mentioned difficulties coping with their own grief, particularly when the patient was young or when life supports were withdrawn," the survey report finds. They also described "being unsure about how much of their own personal reactions to share with the families, and whether the display of emotions would be interpreted as unprofessional behavior or would imply poor judgment or guilt to the family."

This apprehension sounds lamentably similar to the young physician who was chastised for sharing his patient's cake. How sad that the clinical culture has so blinded doctors to the feelings of their patients' families. Who would object, after their loved one died, to a doctor who shows grief? Would a display of emotion reveal incompetence and unprofessionalism? Or would it evidence compassion, signifying that even a clinician who sees death all the time recognizes that this patient was a unique human being whose dying is a loss to the world?

"We were struck that personal reactions to the death were rarely reviewed," the report's authors conclude, "leaving the staff alone with their occasionally gnawing concerns about proper care and their often strong emotional reactions to the loss."

THERE IS THE COMPLETE RECIPE: From the beginning of their training to the decades of their long careers, medical professionals are not taught to treat dying. Instead, they are hardened to it. The laudable scientific emphasis of their profession focuses them on treatments and cures at the expense of compassionate care. And the emotional isolation they experience, despite encountering intense human difficulties every day, forces them to seek numbness and withdrawal—when that is the opposite of what patients and families need and desire and deserve.

What does this recipe produce? The most cogent answer is probably that of Dr. John Wennberg, whose encyclopedic studies of health-care spending patterns are mentioned in Chapter 4. Three of his findings offer especially cogent conclusions about the gap between practitioners and patients in end-of-life care.

First, there is great variation across the country in how much medical care these patients receive, and the differences between one region and another are determined by the supply of hospital beds and physicians, not by "patients' preferences or the rate of illness."

Second, people who live where the most medicine is applied to their care "do not seem to have better outcomes." Rather, a higher number of hospital beds means only that people are admitted sooner and stay longer in intensive care.

Third—and most incredible of all—instead of more medical treatment leading to longer lives for patients, the opposite happens. In regions where there are fewer doctors and hospital beds, "patients at the end of life tend to have lower mortality and do better on other measures of quality." Meanwhile, increased treatment "was associated with worse outcomes. Mortality was between two percent and five percent higher, possibly because greater use of hospital and specialist care exposes populations to greater risks of medical errors."

The implications of these findings are enormous. What Wennberg is saying, in essence, is that for patients who are dying slowly of advanced illness, using more medical care could actually shorten their life.

CLEARLY THAT IS THE OPPOSITE of what health-care providers intend. This book's final chapter details how medical education, state and federal laws, and consumer demands can make a huge difference in the quality of end-of-life care in America. Doctors and nurses could be powerful allies.

As a halfway measure, some educators of physicians concede that palliative and hospice principles may be useful to doctors practicing general medicine but that surgeons and other specialists do not need training in care of the dying. The Institute of Medicine has considered this argument. Based on the premise that death is a universal aspect of the human condition, the institute answers: "Every health professional who deals directly with patients and families needs a basic grounding in dealing competently and compassionately with seriously ill and dying patients."

The institute could have gone further. After all, caring for the dying brings medicine's commendable scientific powers into better balance with its humane mission. Applying that shift in a sweeping manner, all across health care, could positively reorient everything from how vaccines are given to when appointments are scheduled, from where doctors' offices are located to the color of the walls in hospital rooms. The potential for improving the patient's and family's experience should not be limited merely to those in an extreme condition. Is there any facet of health care today that suffers from an excess of attention to the emotional needs of patients?

Maybe at some future time medicine will have to reckon with that welcome problem. Until then, patients seeking a humanizing influence on medical technology will rely heavily on their families. Indeed, they will need the support of their loved ones more than ever—to advocate on their behalf, to insist on attention, to help make hard decisions. Until hospitals and nursing homes improve dramatically in their management of pain, for example, there will be no substitute for a family member standing in a hallway and loudly demanding relief for their loved one.

This new role for family members—caring for parents, spouses, and siblings who are dying slowly—is not easy. It requires a huge sacrifice of time. It can be backbreakingly expensive. It can test their loyalty like never before.

Yet many families are also discovering remarkable gifts in providing end-of-life care, an intimacy and richness without equal in their lives. As the next chapter shows, the shared courage and powerful bond between a person on life's last journey and family members easing that path can create nothing less than a new kind of love.

AS FOR ABBY DONALDSON, the student engrossed in cadaver dissection, she is now in her last year of medical school. She plans to practice pediatrics because she likes its emphasis on preventing illness rather than treating it, and because she loves "the positive attitude of children."

After her gross anatomy final exam, Abby wanted to go back to the lab to say good-bye to her cadaver. But she had another test looming and had to study. By the time she was free, the remains had been removed.

"I was really disappointed. I would have liked to sit in the corner and let the humanness come in again. I feel like I missed that opportunity."

At the end of the year the school held a memorial service for body donors, after which their ashes were sent to their families. Abby found herself making a speech at the event.

"I spoke about how the gross anatomy experience both initiated us into clinical medicine and galvanized our class into a group of people who will never be able to return the knowledge gained—the intimate knowledge of the human body."

Quite apart from the academic lessons, Abby says, some of the emotional experience resurfaced in her subsequent contact with patients. But now it takes a different form.

"The access to the human body that I felt so acutely during gross anatomy is echoed in the access to the emotions, fears, and concerns that are expressed by the living patients I have seen," she says.

The other way Abby has worked to keep her education in perspective is by writing about it. First she kept a journal, then she wrote essays.

Eventually she penned poems about the experience of dissecting that cadaver, the woman whose name she never learned.

In her writing Abby wonders if the woman's husband would object to what students did with her body. Abby also assigns emotions to parts of the body, with muscles being stubborn and organs vulnerable. The naked reality of dissection becomes garbed in metaphor.

Why poems? To document her sensibility. To set down that innocence as an artifact of what she was like at the moment her doctoring life began.

"It seemed to me," Abby says, "that some day, when I had been working in medicine for years, I would appreciate being able to look back at what I was thinking when I first started out. I hope it will be refreshing for me to sort of reexperience that wonder at some point in the future."

Wonder. How admirable it sounds, how humble and optimistic. And, throughout her skilled but flawed profession, how needed.

"Somehow it is comforting," Abby writes in one poem, "that there is beauty too, in this skinless, headless, death-cold body lying naked-hollow on the cold silvery metal. For the first time: beauty."

PART FOUR

MEDICINE AND LOVE ARE NOT THE SAME THING

Passing through the gates of death is like passing quietly through the gate in a pasture fence. On the other side, you keep walking, without the need to look back. No shock, no drama, just the lifting of a plank or two in a simple wooden gate in a clearing. Neither pain, nor floods of light, nor great voices, but just the silent crossing of a meadow.

—MARK HELPRIN

We sometimes congratulate ourselves at the moment of waking from a troubled dream; it may be so the moment after death.

—NATHANIEL HAWTHORNE

CHAPTER SEVENTEEN

ONE EXPERIENCE

On December 12, 2003, John Williams of Chula Vista, California, rose with the sun. He spent some time that early morning putting his affairs in order. Although he was in good health, John had recently made arrangements with a local funeral home. He put several envelopes on the kitchen counter detailing his retirement funds and bank accounts. One envelope was addressed to the adult son of his wife of two decades, Eiko.

The sixty-eight-year-old man walked outside his three-bedroom home on Blackwood Road. The yard and gardens were well maintained, as always. Then he drove to Sharp Chula Vista Medical Center, a 330-bed hospital in the South Bay area near San Diego.

John knew the way well. He had been driving that route for months while his wife battled lung cancer. Eiko, seventy-four, had received chemotherapy and radiation. But she suffered a blood clot at home and landed in intensive care.

By all accounts, John Williams was a devoted husband. He visited his wife so often, he knew the ICU staff and doctors by name.

That Friday morning he had a quiet early visit with his wife. Then staffers asked him to leave the room while they provided some care to Eiko. John went outside, but only for a few minutes. When he returned he followed his routine of walking up to the hospital's security guard and showing him the identification required for entry. John reached his wife's room for the second time at about eight A.M.

In some ways it had already been a long day.

While the ICU staff stood at a nursing station about twenty feet away, John Williams pulled out a .38-caliber revolver. He pressed the barrel against his wife's chest, just below the breast, and fired. Eiko died instantly. Then he stepped back, placed the gun over his own heart, and pulled the trigger. He lingered only a few minutes.

Authorities say about 750 such mercy killings occur in America each year. There is nothing merciful about murder. But the only alternative may be prolonged torture, physical and emotional pain without relief, despair of recovery, and the indignity of overly invasive medical care.

This is not to say that Sharp Chula Vista Hospital was doing a bad job for Eiko, at least according to current medical values. Perhaps her situation justified aggressive intervention at that moment. Confidentiality of medical records, while appropriate, makes it impossible to know. Since she had lung cancer, a slow terminal illness, it is fair to ask why Eiko was in intensive care so long that her husband knew the staff. ICUs are excellent for patients in crisis or those experiencing trauma such as a car accident. ICUs are not designed for a person with an incremental disease. They do not provide care tailored to the particular needs of the individual human being who is dying gradually and irreversibly. Think of it as simply as this: There is no music playing; there is no art on the walls.

Why would 750 people every year decide that death for their loved ones was a merciful escape from the foreseeable medical options? The only possible answer is that they cannot bear to watch their loved ones suffer. They act on a violent combination of compassion and despair.

Mercy killings are an aberration, but the emotions behind them are not. Rather, they represent the most dire expression of what thousands of families in America now face more quietly every day. They see their incrementally dying loved ones lying in hospitals—health professionals at the bedside unschooled in end-of-life care, medicine seeking cures long past any such opportunity, clinical interventions intensifying the pain rather than relieving it. Or they see loved ones decaying in nursing homes, their days spent underfed, their pain ignored, their spirit crushed by boredom, their bedsores spreading. People witness all this, and they experience a new form of familial agony.

As more deaths occur because of incremental illnesses, families are thrust into dilemmas for which they have no preparation. How do they decide when medical treatment has become futile, and perhaps contrary to the patient's ultimate interests? How do they know when stopping treatment is cruelty and when it is merciful? How do they apply their loved ones' values when healthy to their predicament while dying? How do they avoid letting their own biases overcome the patient's wishes? How do they reconcile the spiritual event before them with the practical questions it raises? How do they make sure not to confuse medical care with love?

CHAPTER EIGHTEEN

FAMILIES AS "PROBLEMS"

G radual dying presents families with as many challenges as opportunities. Because the majority of people's lives today end in hospitals and nursing homes, it's problematic that those institutions rarely have programs or systems in place to consider the needs of people other than the patient. Nor is it easy for doctors and nurses to recognize how their intentions might conflict with the priorities of family members.

Sometimes it even seems as if families and medical professionals are dealing with different realities. Clinicians' sensible priorities for a patient and families' legitimate emotional needs can directly contradict each other. That was the situation for the wife and children of Conrad Stannus.

Conrad was one of twelve children, a star student and athlete who built a career in the heady New York investment world. He married Suzanne Hilleary, a music producer, and they had two sons. The family lived a hardworking but charmed life.

Then Conrad contracted Waldenstrom's macroglobulinemia, a bone-marrow and blood disease that is extremely rare and always fatal. He underwent chemotherapy, radiation, a bone-marrow transplant with one of his sisters. Those steps slowed the disease, but there was no chance that it would stop.

When Conrad's immune system failed, the team treating him at Mount Sinai Hospital in New York City put him in an isolation tent to protect him from exposure to germs. His sons, Trevor and Samson, were two and three years old. But doctors told Suzanne not to take the children into the tent.

"They said he couldn't touch the kids," she recalled. "I said, 'He's dying anyway. Does it matter if these kids bring something in? So what?'"

For the hospital, it was not a question of recovery but of extending Conrad's life for as long as possible—and learning more about his disease. During that effort the basketball player and skier dropped to 113 pounds.

"He looked Biafran, he looked HIV-positive," Suzanne said. "Contrary to what the doctors were worried about, I believe those kids were keeping him alive."

Conrad lingered in various stages of illness for years without his sons' infecting him. He also continued to receive aggressive medical interventions, over Suzanne's protests that these efforts were futile and dehumanizing. She suspected that the doctors were motivated more by their research interest than by wanting to help the patient. Eventually Conrad contracted pneumonia. Suzanne arrived one day to discover he had received a tracheotomy—a cut in his throat for inserting a breathing tube. He would be on a ventilator for the rest of his life. She was livid.

"The doctors said they wanted to gain him extra time. I said, 'Extra time for what?'"

Because Conrad could no longer speak, Suzanne arranged for him to have a laptop computer close at hand. When he had the energy, he would type e-mails to his sons. The final weeks were turbulent, with constant clashes between Suzanne and the medical team. When Conrad became comatose—"not moving, atrophied, emaciated" is Suzanne's description—she finally persuaded the team to disconnect his breathing support. He received medication to minimize any discomfort.

"I made them take all the machines out," she said. "They still insisted on monitors so they could watch from the hall."

Conrad died on April 12, 2000. His sons were seven and six. Despite the isolation tent, they knew their father well. They still have those e-mails, too.

DIFFERENT REALITIES: What made sense for the medical team was to keep the patient in sterile circumstances, to prolong his life as long as possible. The merits of this thinking are obvious. For family members, the problem was not that the doctors were unreasonable. They simply felt that clinical priorities were outweighed by a larger emotional truth: Children need to know their father before he dies.

Such clashes are far from rare. A Duke University study interviewed

ICU patients and their families, as well as the doctors and nurses who cared for them, and found conflict in 78 percent of the cases.

The most common area of controversy was whether to withdraw or maintain a particular treatment. Three-quarters of those cases involved medical staff who wanted to continue treatment aggressively when the family did not.

The second area of debate was about medical tasks that were less consequential but still important, such as how much pain medication a patient should receive. There were many communication problems, too, whether the issue was a family not feeling fully informed, or a doctor not being able to discuss care decisions with a family that did not speak English. Sometimes conflict occurred because family members rarely visited the patient yet insisted upon all possible life-extending measures.

There were also clashes within families, the Duke study found. "There was a lot of baggage they came in with," one clinician told researchers. Rather than providing a means for expressing the patients' wishes and values, treatment choices became "a forum for control issues, as in who was gonna make what decision and who proves to mom that they loved her more."

Sometimes conflict is healthy, of course. If the medical system applies its scientific knowledge and expertise and the family exerts its empathy and grief, the two forces are bound to rub up against each other. This strife could conceivably create a positive scenario, as the strengths of each side combine for an ideal outcome.

While this rosy possibility sometimes does occur, the opposite is vastly more common. If you put people in a heightened emotional state into an environment where they have little sense of control, and then you give expert strangers all the power, you have a recipe for conflict. The resulting suffering is indisputable. In one study measuring the quality of care in different settings, families reported that their loved ones who were in a hospital or nursing home did not receive adequate help with pain and breathing difficulties, obtained insufficient emotional support, and in general were treated with less respect.

Those findings echo other studies of end-of-life care but have the unique perspective of coming from witnesses: people who stand at nursing stations shouting for more pain drugs for their mother, who pace and wring their hands while their panicked spouse gasps for breath. These people not only are grieving the loss that is happening before their eyes—itself a powerful and unfamiliar experience—but also are struggling with decisions of dizzying ethical complexity that bear consequences more permanent than any they may have encountered before.

Their woes are exacerbated by the fact that the very people they turn to for guidance and support view them as "problems." One survey asked legal and medical staffers at New York City hospitals what created the most conflict in end-of-life care. "Nearly everyone declared 'families,'" reports the findings in the *Annals of Internal Medicine*. "One physician's response was typical: 'They're too emotional. They don't understand what's going on.'"

Families of patients who have died after suffering at the hands of a callous medical system might gladly stand in line to wring that physician's neck. The problem is not one doctor, however, but an entire system of care that sees an obstacle in what is actually a resource.

Today families represent arguably the fastest-growing component of health care. Many patients who a decade ago would have stayed in the hospital for a week after a surgery now go home the same day. Family members make this cost containment possible by changing dressings, giving medications, taking vital signs. At the end of a person's life this shift is particularly acute. The demands on spouses and children can become all-involving, twenty-four hours a day, bringing exhaustion, caregiver illnesses, even bankruptcy.

More broadly, the doctor's derision of families as "too emotional" also shows a misunderstanding about who the health system is for—patients, not physicians; their families rather than nurses and technicians. It is about care, not convenience. The emotional behavior of family members at the end of a patient's life is evidence of nothing more than their humanity and sometimes provides a useful indicator of what the patient needs.

"Institutional and reimbursement policies, lack of time, and regulatory oversight are often barriers to meaningful attempts to engage and support families," continues the *Annals of Internal Medicine* article. "A persistent tendency is evident, in both the literature and the practice of health care delivery, to equate families with trouble."

Perhaps this equation occurs because families themselves are so troubled when their loved ones are dying.

"Physical changes do cause many emotional difficulties for . . . family and friends," write longtime hospice nurses Maggie Callanan and Patricia Kelley. "When a father becomes incontinent and his son must clean and change him . . . when a husband can no longer brush his teeth and his wife must moisten his dry, sticky mouth . . . when a brother is in pain and his sister must give him medicine . . . these occasions can demonstrate great love. They can also generate great pain, and lead to many feelings and questions more difficult to cope with than physical needs.

"When someone you love is dying, you'll always be dealing with sadness. But your response to that sadness depends on many elements, often related to your previous experience with death. If you haven't had much experience, or haven't had role models who showed you how to behave around dying people, how can you manage?"

CERTAINLY EXPERIENCE HELPS. But most families would rather provide good care when it is needed than discover too late how they might have done better. Thus, managing a loved one's illness demands more than experience. It requires a health system that accepts how dying has changed and recognizes that the sick person is not the only one who needs help.

"Trying to keep a full-time job going and take care of Bob was a major, major stress," recalled Ann Beauchamp of Bel Air, Maryland. "There was no support whatsoever. There was no social worker asking me how it was going. I was totally on my own."

When Ann married Bob in 1989, he already had Crohn's disease. To control that illness, which affects the intestines, he'd taken the steroid prednisone for nearly two decades. "It is a short-term miracle drug," Ann said, "but it's a long-term disaster."

The first problems were colitis flare-ups. Bob started missing days at the bank where he and Ann worked. One time when he returned after a few days out, Bob's supervisor asked if he had considered going out on disability. Reluctantly, he accepted the reality that he could not be a dependable employee until his health stabilized.

That was the hope. Instead, Bob's downward spiral was under way. It lasted ten years.

The steroid treatment led to problems with his joints. That made him less active, resulting in weight gain and eventually, with further steroid side effects, adult-onset diabetes. As Bob lost sensation in his feet, needing canes to walk and becoming unable to drive, his dependence on Ann grew.

"With chronic disease, on any given day you don't see a decline," Ann said. "But if you look back six months, you can make a list of things that are lost. Like he can't do the dishes now, because he can't stand. He used to come downstairs twice a day. Then once a day. Then once every few days. The dreams get taken away piece by piece."

The strains were not only medical. "We were in a tight financial situation," Ann said. "The insurers told us, 'Don't worry, you'll get all your back payments when it's approved.' Well, great, but what about the rent this month?"

In 1996 Bob developed leg ulcers. That meant several trips weekly to a wound-care center, a logistical impossibility for a woman with a full-time job. "I had to watch every minute of leave time, because I could only take so much sick time for a family member per year."

Managing Bob's care was a lonely business, Ann recalled. "Bob's parents are deceased, and my family is three states away. I started looking for a job that was flexible, so if I missed time for an appointment, I could make up the time. I was at one law firm and it didn't work out. You know, 'You came in at 9:03.'"

Their sex life changed as well. "The last time we were about to . . . well, with all the inactivity and immobility, he was over four hundred pounds. Plus his hips were so bad. We weren't able to make the connection. We improvised. And certainly the kissing and affection was there. We would tell each other dozens of times a day that we loved each other. But it was hard, hard on us both."

Ann began to burn out. "Nobody ever suggested respite services or anything like that. I was totally alone, always alone."

Ann did try the employee-assistance program at work. "The counselor said, 'I don't know why you don't just give up.' I told her: 'I've given up my career aspirations. I've given up on having a family. I've given up on my church activities. It's not like I'm going to abandon my husband. In sickness and in health, there are some people who do sign up for life.'"

In late 2001 Bob's decline accelerated. He and Ann decided to take a risk. He would undergo gastric-bypass surgery, otherwise known as stomach stapling. With his weight reduced, they would be able to address his other problems. "It was a last-ditch act of desperation. Or maybe it was suicide-by-doctor. We didn't really talk about [whether this would] kill him. I don't think Bob realized what all the implications were. Me, I was expecting it to be a nightmare summer."

Bob's surgery began later than scheduled, so Ann was at work. When she arrived at the hospital, there was no provision whatsoever for helping a family member. "I was there for three hours, and I didn't even know where I was supposed to be waiting. At about two A.M. they told me he was in the surgical ICU, and I got to see him."

Bob suffered complications from the surgery, requiring many follow-up procedures. "Day after day I'm at work, and I'd give consent over the phone," Ann recalled. "I couldn't drop my whole life and hang out at the ICU. I couldn't afford a leave of absence."

Even if that had been an option, she said, the nightly visits curbed her enthusiasm for waiting around. The problem was not a lack of love but an excess of solitude.

"Cooling my heels in a hospital waiting room, those are very long hours when you're the only one there. One night leaving, when there had been a whole family camped out for someone else there, in the elevator I thought, 'Well, Bob, you've just had one more visitor than I'll ever have.'"

When Ann arrived at the hospital after work that Monday, a physician was waiting for her in the hallway. "I think it was to keep me from going in the room. But also, then you know it's serious, because doctors don't just hang out like that."

The doctor delivered the news that Bob's heart had stopped twice since four-thirty that afternoon. Because there was no signed order in place to the contrary, the medical staff had restarted his heart both times. The next few hours only reinforced how little the hospital was equipped to treat anyone other than Bob.

"They're telling me about making decisions, and they keep asking, 'Is there any other family member that can be here?'" Ann answered repeatedly that it was just her. Gradually she realized what no one had shown the courage to put into words. "I'm going to have to tell them to let him go. This is going to happen tonight.

"I went in to say good-bye. While I was in there his heart stopped. The team comes rushing in. After, one of them said, 'We can do this all night.' I thought, why? Why would you do this?

"The doctor came over and read me a list of all the organ failures. I asked, 'Are we sustaining his life or prolonging it?' The doctor never actually said, 'He's dying.' I asked again. He goes down the list again. I said, 'Let him go. The next time his heart stops, let him go.' Then I went into the room.

"It took only a few minutes. The line goes horizontal. The ventilator is still going, his chest is going up and down, but he's not there anymore. It was a scene out of a horror movie, and I was totally alone.

"The technician came in after a few minutes and switched off the machine. They said, 'Is there anybody we should call?' No, it's only me.

"I wandered back to the nurses' station. What do I do now? What forms do I have to fill out?"

Dazed, Ann made her way to the parking garage, drove home, left a voice message for her boss, and sent an e-mail to friends and family.

"The next morning my boss calls up. She's a young widow who lost her husband to AIDS from a transfusion. She says, 'We're taking you to lunch.' I tell her I have to be at the funeral home. She says, 'We're coming with you.' Thank God they did. I was in a total daze. Who knows what I would have said yes to? They took me to an Italian restaurant and made sure my wineglass didn't stay empty."

In retrospect, Ann finds no fault with the medical treatment Bob received. The problem was the system's insensitivity to the effect that gradual dying has on people close to the patient.

After eighteen months of self-imposed solitude, Ann began dating again. Now forty-nine, she recently met a widower whose wife died two years previously. They are moving slowly, she said. "We both know that we're healing." Then she laughed. "Eleven years of pent-up sexual frustration has worked itself out. He was, I'm sure, the happy recipient of that."

Though she is proud of her current job as an administrative assistant at the Space Telescope Science Institute in Baltimore, Ann's experience with Bob led her back to school. She enrolled in Loyola College's master's program in pastoral counseling.

"I was talking with so many widows, I thought: I could get paid to do this. In fact, I got a divinity degree twenty years ago, so this will bring everything full circle.

"It is good to be back into theology, the caring side. And now I'll know a little about what I'm doing. Especially when I'm working with people who are suffering."

CHAPTER NINETEEN

NO ONE IN CHARGE

The obvious solution is to have a big family, preferably nearby. However, manufacturing supportive siblings is rather hard on short notice. The resource of an extended family within driving range is not as common as it once was, now that Americans on average have fewer children, move every six years, and change careers every seven. Almost one-sixth of the U.S. population, some 43 million people, changes its location annually. In a wholesale reversal of pre–World War II family patterns, rare is the household today with multiple generations under one roof.

Still, the mobility that enables people to leap the continent for a better job sometimes also allows travel to help care for a seriously ill loved one. Federal laws require employers to keep jobs open for months while employees care for sick family members—assuming that workers can afford the time without pay. So, with today's light-footed and responsive society, there remains a fair chance that people near the end of life will have family members helping with their care.

Unfortunately, the complexity of decisions these families face might make some of them long for Ann Beauchamp's solitude. For example, siblings will have divergent relationships with a terminally ill parent, with the remaining healthy parent, with medical science. They may have different religions, different ideas about what constitutes a meaningful life, different support systems in their own lives, different amounts of time available, different other demands on their emotions (such as children), different capacities to absorb the financial strain of providing care, and different ideas about what the patient wants.

Yet in the era of incremental illness, these family members are routinely called upon to make consensus decisions of incredible weight and complexity. Does attaching a feeding tube sustain life or prolong torture? Is using a ventilator on a person with respiratory failure an act of hope or denial? When a person is lost in the maze of dementia, is the onset of pneumonia a catastrophe or a mercy?

There are no right answers, no formulas that families can apply to make perfect decisions. Besides, even a perfect answer brings little satisfaction, since whatever they choose the person they love will be gone in the end. Ideally, families should have someone to turn to for help, a guide who understands both the medical situation and the values and preferences of the patient and family.

To that end, some hospitals now offer consultations in "clinical ethics"—discussions with doctors, nurses, and possibly clergy. These sessions educate families about what is going on clinically, informing them about treatment options. Done right, the process identifies potential decisions in the days ahead so that families can make choices in an atmosphere of calm deliberation rather than grieving panic.

Despite the best intentions of its practitioners, however, this work is in its infancy. More often, researchers report and families confirm, people are left floundering, struggling to care for patients who are extremely ill, striving to help them live their remaining days free of suffering. For these families, the medical system is an impediment to a dignified passage. And the experience of dealing with that system can leave a dark bruise that takes years to heal.

ADYN EUGENE SCHUYLER SR. OF EVANSTON, Illinois, was attending the 1939 winter carnival in Memphis when he met Minnie Maude McMullen—the daughter of a cotton-farming judge and "a notorious Southern belle," recalls her daughter Maude Clay of Sumner, Mississippi.

Adyn moved to Mississippi and married his belle. After forty-five years together, in 1984 Minnie began suffering from back pains that were eventually diagnosed as bone cancer. The family cared for her at home.

"My mother died in this house, downstairs in the front bedroom," Maude says. "She had a hard passing. That is not an unpainful illness."

Afterward Adyn "moped around," Maude says. "It was kind of a trial for him."

Adyn's bachelorhood was to last sixteen years, during which he out-lived one girlfriend, then found himself another. There were signs that time was catching up with him, problems with his balance and misplaced credit cards. Adyn relished his independence, though, particularly driv-ing. That worried his family terribly. "We thought he was a lawsuit wait-ing to happen, if he goes and hits anyone," Maude recalls. The year he turned ninety-one, Adyn bought himself the latest in his lifetime string of new big Buicks—his only concession to age being that this one was not a convertible.

When his license expired, Maude says, "we thought that would be a natural end to it, and we'll just not renew it." He kept asking for help re-newing the license; Maude stalled. Adyn decided to go on his own.

"Now there's two women up there who do the tests," Maude says. "Both my teenagers, these women flunked them. Not coming to a com-plete stop or something like that. So, I thought again, that'll do it."

Three hours later Adyn returned, and Maude prepared herself. "This will be depressing for him, probably."

Instead, he'd passed. "Those women couldn't have been nicer," she remembers him saying. "A license costs twenty dollars and I only had five, so they loaned me the fifteen dollars, too."

Maude laughs at the memory. "I was out of my league. I thought they were going to fail him, and instead he charmed the pants off of them."

Soon after that little victory, Adyn's previously minor health problems worsened. He fell, broke his leg, suffered two minor strokes. The family moved him into a graduated-care facility and hired a man to drive Adyn to his girlfriend's house or out to lunch.

The family gave Adyn a panic button alarm, too, so he could call for help in an emergency. He used it nearly a dozen times, after one fall or an-other. The facility's medic team would come quickly, but he set strict lim-its on their assistance. "He insisted that he not go to the hospital," Maude says. The medics always gave in. "He was a very forceful person, even though he was this tiny thing at the end."

Adyn was also determined to turn aside any conversation about the medical care he wanted at the end of his life. "He wouldn't have it with us. 'Whatever you kids want to do is fine with me.'"

Maude, her brother, Adyn Jr., and her sister Shelley accepted that an-swer. "We didn't have the guts," Maude recalls, "or the mental power, or whatever it takes to transfer the power, to stop being the kids and become the ones in charge. We didn't say, 'Here's a living will, now sign it.'"

One night in May 2004—Adyn was ninety-two by then—he had a fall that the rapid-response team considered more serious. "To this day I wonder if it was something as simple as food poisoning," Maude says. "But the medic people decided that's it, it was their professional duty to take him to the emergency room."

Maude arrived at the hospital about ten-thirty to find Adyn his usual polite self. "Every time he was going to throw up he would say, 'Maude, you're going to have to leave the room. I'm having a delicate moment.'"

A doctor admitted Adyn to the hospital, though he was not moved to a room until 5:30 A.M. Maude went home to ready her children for school. When she returned at ten, "he was almost dead. I hadn't known it was so severe. No one could figure out what happened. They sent him down for a sonogram to see if he had a blockage."

On the way Maude asked her father if he needed anything. "'Just you,' he said, and he squeezed my hand," she recalls, tearing up at the memory. "That was really our last communication."

Emergency exploratory surgery might have found the problem, Maude says, "but this one doctor said Daddy was in such a weakened condition, he couldn't even do that. He said, 'This is a dying man. Do you want comfort measures only?'"

Maude did not want her father to die, but she began to think that his time had come. "The last thing we need to do to him is a bunch of really invasive procedures. He hadn't had the life he loved in a long time." She decided to limit her father's care to comfort only. "I had been taking care of him for the last ten years. I thought I was the person in charge."

Another physician, however, called Shelley. "He told her, 'We don't want to do any more invasive, life-support stuff, right?' And she said, 'Wait a minute, what is life-support stuff?' He said they could take him to intensive care and put him on a respirator. And she said okay, do that."

By that time Adyn Sr. was no longer conscious, but that did not make Maude and her brother any less upset.

"We knew it would do no good," Maude recalls. "It was just going to prolong things. And intensive-care units are harrowing places. They won't let you in there but one hour in the morning and one hour in the afternoon. And the respirator? They stick this thing down your throat, and you are artificially being kept breathing."

The siblings moved into long-standing familial roles. Adyn Jr. was ready to argue with anyone. Shelley, while unafraid to tangle with him, was going through a difficult divorce that heightened her emotions. She also hadn't spent time with her father in months. Maude served as peacemaker and go-between. In the dispute over her father's care, she had her hands full.

"He and she were having these knock-down drag-out fights, going at it ninety to nothing," Maude remembers. "She's saying Daddy's going to get well, we just have to believe. And he's saying, 'You're . . . just feeling guilty 'cause you haven't seen him.' And me, I'm there saying we got to stick to-gether, we're all we have left now."

They argued at the hospital. They debated in the car. They shouted in the family house, which is now Maude's home. "One night he said he was going to go stay at a hotel because my sister was here."

One of Adyn Sr.'s old hunting and fishing friends had been the local Episcopal minister before going on to a church leadership position in Arkansas. He came to the hospital and gave Adyn last rites. He said his old friend would not have wanted to endure struggling for breath on a machine.

That guidance seemed to ease tensions somewhat, Maude recalls. So did a pulmonologist's candor a day later. "He told us that there was a one percent chance that our daddy would pull out of this. And if he did, he would be a complete vegetable. At that point even my sister said okay."

The family informed the medical team that they were prepared for the respirator to be removed. By then both Adyn Jr. and Maude had said good-bye to their father. "We did it alone, at the bedside," Maude says. "We told him how much we loved him.

"But my sister, she had this whole thing going because she hadn't seen him since Easter and now this was June. She goes in there. It was very sad to me to watch. And she told him that it was okay for him to die. Maybe what she said, that was his last thing, because there had been one person still hanging on to him. But she had finally come to terms with her-self and with the situation. Daddy would be so much worse if he survived. So she had just given him permission to die."

The three siblings crowded into the room together, accompanied by a local minister. Then they went to meet with their father's doctors and hos-pital administrators, leaving one nurse and the pastor in Adyn's room.

At the meeting a senior physician promptly told the family that Adyn did not meet the criteria for disconnecting a respirator. Maude cannot re-call what the reason might have been. "It's gone to that place where I'd have to be hypnotized to find it."

She remembers quite clearly, however, being livid. "There is a ninety-two-year-old father in there and a pulmonary specialist says a one percent chance of being at most a vegetable, and he is saying that we as a hospital do not have the authority to do this. He started on this religious thing, and he's really talking to my sister. 'It is wrong to take a life.' My brother and I are going, 'It is wrong to keep him alive. It is racking him out and it is racking us out.'"

The doctor held firm; the respirator would not be removed. But his stance had an unexpected effect.

"That was a force that brought us back together," Maude says. "There was now an interloper. . . . We all realized that our common enemy was not ourselves, but this hospital."

Adyn Jr. lost his temper. "My brother was roaring up: 'If I can't do this, I will sue this hospital for everything.' And he goes, 'There's nothing that says I can't take him out of here right now, no law that I can't just put him in a wheelchair and go.'"

At that moment the intensive-care nurse interrupted the meeting with the news that Adyn Sr. had died.

"My brother kind of laughed, he did. He told those hospital administrators that Daddy always did have a way of getting in the last word."

They held a high Episcopal funeral, conducted by Adyn's friend. Settling the estate required the siblings to speak by phone several times, but so far they have not been in the same room together. Maude remains optimistic that the unity they felt on their father's behalf in that hospital meeting will overcome any damage from debating his final care.

"You're not required to love and spend time with your siblings, but it's such a beautiful thing if you can. I'm hoping we'll all realize eventually that we are the only people left from this unit."

THE CHALLENGES OF CARING for a person who is dying are not only emotional. One nationwide survey, of nearly one thousand patients whose primary caregiver was a family member, found burdens that involved money, transportation, household management, pain control, and personal care. People with more of these unmet needs reported a higher economic burden, a higher rate of depression, and a greater likelihood of considering euthanasia or physician-assisted suicide.

Unfortunately, these patients' medical situation was typical for people with incremental illnesses. That is, a majority experienced substantial untreated pain, 18 percent were bedridden most of the day, 71 percent had shortness of breath, 36 percent were to some degree incontinent. In other words, because of the unresponsiveness of the health system to gradual dying, these people had many unmet needs quite apart from issues affecting their families.

The impact on those families was clear and sometimes severe. For patients with many unmet needs, 45 percent of family caregivers said the cost of providing care was "a moderate or great economic hardship." Families reported spending 10 percent of the household income on health-care costs beyond insurance premiums. In addition to caretaking, they therefore had to get additional jobs, sell assets, or take out loans.

Although the survey focused on unmet nonmedical needs, it also found a correlation between those needs and the perceived quality of medical care. In essence, families consistently reported that if the physicians they dealt with listened to their needs, they were less likely to be depressed and less likely to say that their caretaking role interfered with their lives. Conversely, caregivers who found their burdens excessive were more likely to become sick themselves.

The survey's authors draw two salient conclusions. First, if unskilled care became a benefit covered by health insurance, it would improve patients' lives and reduce their demands on costly skilled providers like doctors and nurses. Second, doctors can lighten the burden on families without incurring extra costs, "simply by listening well."

One study in Oregon—interviewing patients before their death and loved ones afterward—concludes that shortcomings in communication were the primary reason families were dissatisfied with end-of-life care.

"Persons with life-threatening illnesses indicated that health professionals focus on medical and physical interventions, give too little information, appear uncomfortable talking about death, and do not include family members in conversations," the report says. In focus-group sessions, the report continues, "caregivers report exhaustion. They said that doctors do not appreciate the impact of the illness on their lives and rarely consult them, although all treatment decisions affect them."

That these views were insufficiently respected is telling, the survey says, given the level of family engagement in the situation. Caregivers frequently referred to "our illness," for example, reflecting the impact of the patient's sickness on their lives. Families said they knew their loved one best and willingly put their lives on hold in order to help. That makes being excluded from decision making especially hard to accept.

As for families whose loved one had died, the study finds, "bereaved persons wish that physicians would tell families when the end is near, and avoid interrupting the process of dying with medical and often futile tasks."

They said the last days of their loved one's life were highly meaningful, yet they described "frequent disregard for patient/family wishes" in terms of limiting care. That gap raises a serious ethical question about who ought to be in charge of patient decisions, and who actually is.

COMMUNICATION PROBLEMS are more than awkward conversations or dialogues that don't take place. Poor communication interferes with the most basic ingredient of health-care decision making—an exchange of information—and in the heightened atmosphere of a possible loved one's death, mistakes are of ultimate consequence.

The Meenan family's experience proves this point in excruciating slow motion.

Francis Meenan was a lifelong New Yorker whose father had come by ship from Ireland. Three of his brothers were New York City policemen, and Francis drove a city bus. Though his father had pulled him from school in the tenth grade to work, Francis obtained his GED on the G.I. Bill and remained a lifelong advocate of education. He married Maureen, fathered six children—Kevin, Colleen, Tara, Maura, Peggy, and Michael— and was a demanding taskmaster of them.

He had also contracted rheumatic fever as a teenager. That illness attacks the heart's valves, but Francis led a healthy and active life.

"Then one Father's Day when he was about thirty-five, I walked into the bathroom to find him coughing up pints of blood," recalls Kevin, who was thirteen at the time. "I thought he was going to die then."

Emergency surgery replaced Francis's damaged mitral valve with the same valve from a pig's heart—which closely resembles the human anatomy and can last up to twenty years. Francis spent more than a month in the hospital.

"The first time I saw him on a respirator, with a dozen tubes connected to him, that was a very traumatic moment," Kevin says. "Hearing that they sawed open all of his ribs, and seeing his scar—half the width of a sausage, from his trachea to his belly button—very traumatic."

But Francis recovered, living another fifteen years before his aortic valve failed. "When he learned that, his comment was that he would rather die than have the surgery, the pain he encountered the first time was so traumatic," Kevin says.

Francis's doctor persuaded him to have exploratory surgery instead, and he was given a bed beside an eighty-year-old man who was on his feet the day after open-heart surgery. Francis assumed the science had progressed, agreed to the operation, and was walking himself in a day or two.

In 1996, twenty-nine years after Francis's initial surgery, the first pig valve began to fail. His situation typified recent progress in medicine; a few years earlier he would simply have died. Instead, Francis lived to see his children fulfill his commitment to education—they not only attended Catholic grade school and high school, as he had hoped, they obtained four graduate degrees among them. His children were nurses, a lawyer, an investment banker, and more. Francis also lived to see them married, to know his grandchildren, to celebrate a decades-longer marriage to Maureen.

Francis's extra years embodied the gains of twentieth-century medicine; later they also revealed how medicine has not changed to cope with the results of that success. To begin with, this time the operation was more dangerous.

"He was in such a fragile state, and this was to be his fourth open-heart surgery," Kevin recalls. "Every subsequent surgery is that much more risky than the previous one. They told him there was a thirty percent chance that he would not survive."

The alternative was no better, though. Francis by then had advanced congestive heart failure. His lungs were filling with fluid; he was always short of breath. Kevin remembers: "His doctor said, 'If you don't have the valve replacement, you'll probably be dead within six months. And it will not be a comfortable passing.'"

Francis decided to have the operation at Columbia-Presbyterian Hospital in Manhattan. The entire family gathered before the procedure.

"We walked him to those last couple doors, before the operating room," Kevin says. "He looked up at the seven of us, and he said, 'I am so proud of all of you guys.' And with that, they wheeled him in. At that point we were all crying."

The surgery, expected to last four or five hours, took almost nine. Francis went into a coma. It lasted one hundred days.

On day two several family members were in the room when nurses were cleaning Francis, and they saw a wound on his buttock. "We said, 'What the heck is that?'" Kevin says.

It was a burn. "When they shocked his heart back after the surgery, he was on a metal table, of course, and they usually have a pad to ground you. That malfunctioned. The poor guy is in a coma, and he wound up with a second-degree burn the size of a small football. That wound eventually caused as much discomfort and pain as the heart surgery itself."

It also caused a shift in the family's relationship with the medical team. After all, no one had told them about the burn. They asked to see Francis's chart. "We wanted to audit what was happening to him. But the hospital said no. We were denied access to his chart because he did not have a signed health proxy."

The Meenans started keeping a chart of their own. They still have it today, a three-ring binder labeled "Comprehensive Care Plan."

"It was a very frustrating, agonizing experience," Kevin says. "But we were loving our dad, caring for him, and we wanted to do something."

They set up a system of vigilance, eighteen hours a day, with many family members maintaining that schedule for the full hundred days. Such steadfastness made a difference with the nursing team. One nurse even pulled Kevin aside to confide her suspicion that Francis's burn may have been caused by negligence.

The Meenans observed problems with their father's ongoing care, too. It was sophisticated but not managed well—or more accurately, not managed at all. Francis was under treatment by a wound-care team for his incision, a respiratory team dealing with complications from his congestive heart failure, a cardiac team focused on his heart, a renal team after his kidneys failed, a pulmonary team for his ventilator, and a nutritional team for his feeding tube. And all the teams had nothing to do with one another.

"A doctor would walk in with the chart, on rounds, with a couple of residents or students," Kevin remembers. "He would say, 'This is a male patient, sixty-five years old, this complication, that complication.' Our dad was a live case study. Anyway, they'd go through their thing, then Dr. X would call the nurse in. 'The belly's too distended. The blood pressure's too low. Disconnect the feeding through the gastrointestinal tube.'

"We'd hear that, disconnect our dad's food, and we would think, 'Okay, he's the doctor.' Then, an hour and a half later, the nutrition team would show up. They'd say, 'Wait a second. This guy should be getting fed. Restart the feeding tube.'"

The lack of coordination in Francis's care had a gradual effect, Kevin says. "We believed that our dad was at one of the best hospitals in the country. Had he not been at this hospital, he probably would have died. So we felt this was the price to pay, allowing the state of medicine to progress. It was part of the gig.

"As time went on, though, it became more intrusive, more offensive, as they went from day one to day six to day sixty. And during this whole process, we're kind of watching our dad melt away."

Yet the vigil also included touching moments. "One of my more emotional reflections is my mom walking into the room, she'd kiss him, talk to him. And you could see on the monitor there, his pulse would pick up."

The family found inspiration in one of Francis's favorite lines of scripture, from Saint Paul: "I ran the good race. I fought the good fight."

Having medical professionals in the family helped. The nursing sisters and sister-in-law ensured that Francis received bedside care far better than the hospital's busy staff could provide. "It was great watching my sisters walk into the room and spring into nursing mode," Kevin says. "Swabbing his lips, bathing him, massaging his feet. It was comforting and tormenting at the same time."

Eventually the conflicts among doctors and the family's inability to get them to work together on Francis's behalf became "insane," Kevin says. "It was very clear to me that no one is in charge."

He approached a neighbor who attended the same church and whose sons he had coached in basketball. That friend ran a health-care consulting business. Kevin described the doctors' conflicting orders. "He said to me, 'This is the challenge we're trying to teach hospitals about today. They are all struggling with coordination of care.'"

The problem is common: Even excellent doctors with the best of intentions function within health systems that do not acknowledge how dying has changed. Care becomes fragmented, even contradictory.

The situation can leave families angry and frustrated. A study in New York City solicited the views of people who were next of kin to patients who had died in one of five teaching hospitals. Nearly 20 percent of them reported that no doctor was in charge of their loved one's care. Almost half said that although a doctor was in charge, he or she had no relationship to the patient prior to the hospitalization—so the preferences of family and patient were unknown.

As usual for people dying slowly, more than 80 percent of the patients experienced pain, difficulty breathing, or emotional distress. Hospitals' responsiveness to these symptoms "was rated as higher when a physician was seen as clearly in charge," the study finds. Not surprisingly, the worst reports of symptom management—more pain, more difficulty breathing, more distress—came from kin who said no doctor was in charge.

"Symptom control and physician responsiveness to symptoms are serious concerns for hospitalized patients near the end of life and for their families," the study's authors write. "Ensuring that one or more physicians are clearly in charge of each patient may be an important step toward improving the quality of care for hospitalized dying patients."

In other words, the Meenans' anguish was typical. They had an unusual resource, however. Kevin's consultant friend had contacts in the business, among them the chairman of the hospital's board.

"Two hours later the chairman calls," Kevin says. "He said, 'Going forward, Dr. Rose is going to be your go-to guy, your doctor in charge.'" Rose was the cardiac surgeon who had operated on Francis.

It was fortuitous that the Meenans had that connection to help their father. Obviously, the vast majority of people have no such contacts. All they can do is watch and suffer along with their loved one.

At day one hundred, Francis began waking up for short intervals. During his absence the family had celebrated Thanksgiving, Christmas, the New Year. Gradually he woke for longer periods, then he was weaned from the ventilator, then the family was able to feed him.

Francis was still seriously ill, though. The kidney failure meant dialysis three times a week. Congestive heart failure meant a strict diet, with severe limits on fluid intake. He was well enough to go home, but the caretaking was demanding work.

"My sisters would come over and attend to him," Kevin says. "I would go over there and help him out of bed. My wife, Marianne, who is a pediatric intensive-care nurse, he loved for her to massage his feet."

The burn continued to cause problems. "He couldn't lie on his back because of it. He couldn't sit down. He could only lay on one side. It was an indignity on top of the traumatic surgery."

The Meenans sued the hospital over the burn. They had taken photographs of the wound early on, and again when Francis returned home. He gave a deposition as well. The settlement negotiations "were a game of Russian roulette," Kevin says. "The veiled threat was 'we'll hold out till he dies,' because the critical factor in determining a settlement is future-earnings capability and future suffering. It became a perverse dynamic."

The case settled, its details confidential, Kevin says.

Within weeks of returning home, Francis began to decline. He had a rupture at the site in his thigh where the cardiac catheter had been placed during surgery ruptured, causing major blood loss. Then he had trouble breathing, which landed him in the local hospital. The ordeal worsened.

"I went in to visit him at probably eight one morning," Kevin says, "and he had soiled himself. He put his hand down and came up with it on his hand. And he said, 'Kevin, what has happened to me? This is horrible.'

"I went for a nurse, said he needs some help here. I stayed with him till the nurse came in. But then I didn't want to embarrass him by staying, so I left."

That evening his sister Colleen called. Francis was back in a coma and fading rapidly. When his condition stabilized about ten, one daughter took Maureen home. The rest of the family remained at the hospital. His stability faded within the hour.

"By eleven he was mumbling incoherently, he was laboring to breathe. We were trying to communicate, but he wasn't responding. My three sisters, my brother, and myself, we said it looks like he's not going to make it. Should we get Mom or not?"

Then Francis's breathing became extremely difficult, and he began hemorrhaging. They decided that their mother did not need to witness the end. He fought for one breath after another.

The family remembered that line from Saint Paul. "The five of us then were like, 'Dad, stop. Stop. Give up the fight.'"

At 12:30 A.M. that Easter morning, Francis took his last breath and died. The hospital room was quiet at last. The brothers and sisters held one another and cried.

"You ask someone," Kevin reflects, "what were the most memorable moments in your life? I would have to say getting married, your kids being born, and witnessing your mom or dad being like that."

Only in time would family members realize how disorganized their father's care was and how good efforts by individual physicians were not enough to compensate for poor overall coordination. Kevin says the experience had important lessons.

The first is criticism of the health system. "I have a health-care proxy now, and part of that proxy is a do-not-resuscitate order. I don't want to be kept alive for experimental purposes and cause trauma to my family."

The second is a realization about the value of life. "I bet almost ninety percent of the days since my dad got sick, I have worked out. Good health is an unbelievable blessing, and you're supposed to take care of your gifts."

The third lesson is the potential for fulfilling actions that gradual dying provides. "If he had died on the operating table, we would have been denied the opportunity to come together as a family. He and we would never have known that we could come together like that."

To this day Kevin describes his siblings' efforts as heroic. "It was emotional, you bet. But it was a cohesive thing, too, a way to bond that we had never had. And the fact that he was able to come home and have sixty more days, and I was able to sit at his bedside and tell him that I loved him, it was a remarkably positive thing. It deepened my faith."

The final lesson for Kevin is an enduring skepticism about the health system's motives in end-of-life care. "I remember my mom having crates and crates of medical bills. I don't know what the whole cost was, but I bet it was more than a million dollars. Just the ICU, at let's say ten thousand dollars a day with all the care, for one hundred days, that's a million right there.

"To me that's a conflict of interest for the medical people. 'We've got a live guinea pig that we can go to school on.' I wonder, I just wonder, if and when my dad's insurance ran out, whether they would be less motivated to sustain him."

CHAPTER TWENTY

THE ECONOMICS
OF DYING

I t is tempting to dismiss Kevin Meenan's suspicions as the cynicism of
a grieving son. But the financial issues involved in caring for people
who are dying are not so easily set aside.

Although no complete measure of spending on end-of-life care exists,
the Medicare federal health-insurance system provides reliable data for
people who die after turning sixty-five. It is not surprising that people at
the end of their lives incur major health expenses; after all, they usually
are quite sick. Nevertheless, the percentage of Medicare spending devoted to people's final days appears disproportionate.

A 1984 report, for example, found that 5.9 percent of the people eligible for Medicare died during the year being studied. Those people in-
curred 27.9 percent of total Medicare spending.

A 1995 study investigated data from the 2.1 million Americans who
had died in 1987. These people represented 0.9 percent of the U.S. population at the time. Yet medical expenditures on their behalf amounted to
$44.9 billion, about 7.5 percent of the nation's total health-care spending.

When it comes to longevity, American culture affirms that every
penny is well spent if the results are desirable. This society is not the first
that has thought so highly of the value of human life. It is merely the first
economy affluent enough to afford to act on those values.

The spending would make sense if the outcome were desirable. Instead, people suffer needlessly, they receive interventions they do not

want, their lives are prolonged against their wishes. Current policy spends a fortune to achieve ends that people do not seek.

The economic impact is not limited to government's taxpayer-funded programs, either. It reaches further into Americans' wallets. "Chronic and terminal illnesses have serious financial consequences for families," reports the Institute of Medicine. "These financial consequences stem in part from out-of-pocket medical expenses [that is, costs not covered by insurance] but also from lower patient or family income that results from absenteeism, reduced working hours, or job loss related to illness or the demands of caring for an ill family member."

That may be an understatement. The Alexandria, Virginia–based advocacy group Americans for Better Care of the Dying argues that the crushing costs of caring for a dying loved one, as thousands more lives end gradually each year, is creating a new cohort of impoverished senior citizens. Predominantly women—because men on average live shorter lives—these people spend their life savings attempting to provide a dignified final chapter for a loved one. Once the person has died, they discover they have no money left on which to live their remaining days.

Perhaps the definitive study of the financial impact of medical bills came in 2005, in a joint project by the Harvard Medical School and Harvard Law School. Researchers surveyed nearly two thousand bankruptcy filings in five federal courts, interviewing by phone half the people who had filed. They deduced that illness and medical bills were by far the largest reason for personal bankruptcy, causing half of the 1.46 million filings in 2001.

Health insurance offered scant protection against financial calamity: three-quarters of those filing had coverage at the start of the bankrupting illness. Uncovered medical bills of people with insurance averaged $13,460, but the average for people who had cancer was $35,878.

The point merits repetition: Massive spending on end-of-life care would be acceptable if patients were clamoring for ever more treatments and ever greater interventions. Instead, they and their families consistently say they want less heroics and more pain control, less technology and more compassion. The money is all but being wasted.

Ironically, care for the dying is one of those instances in medicine in which spending more does not result in higher quality. Dr. John Wennberg's studies found no correlation between higher spending and reduced mortality or better end-of-life care. But that data only confirms what most people know intuitively. Better care of the irreversibly dying means fewer interventions, less hospitalization, reduced tests and physician office visits—in exchange for dependable at-home nursing care, aggressive pain management, and thorough family support. Such a shift would arguably require less money than the status quo. If the federal government wants to rein in Medicare costs, end-of-life-care expenditures merit close review.

A number of researchers have investigated whether providing hospice care saves money. The answers have been consistently encouraging.

- A 1985 study found that spending for hospice patients in the last month of life is almost one-third less than for people not in hospice.

- A 1995 study found that hospice saved Medicare $1.52 for every dollar spent.

- A 1996 report concluded that hospice saves 25 to 40 percent in the last month of life, and 10 to 17 percent in the last six months of life.

Several studies have found no financial advantage in providing hospice care, but even then there remains the higher quality of care that hospice delivers.

These investigations plumbed Medicare data, a truly national view. A more human-scale example is evident at Virginia Commonwealth University Medical Center in Richmond.

There a local team led by a doctor and a nurse clinical specialist raised money to open a palliative care unit in the hospital. The values and methods of hospice were put to work within the institution's walls—everything from aggressive pain control to therapy dogs, from arts classes to massage. The nonmedical benefits of this approach have already been well documented. But the interesting thing is the difference in cost.

The medical team focused on patients' last five days at the hospital, comparing people in the palliative-care unit with those in regular treatment programs:

- Patients in the palliative care unit required $511 for drugs and chemotherapy; those in the regular hospital required $2,267.

- Lab work for palliative patients was $56; for the others, labs cost $1,134.

- Diagnostic imaging ran $29 for palliative patients, compared with $615 for other patients.

- Medical supplies were $731, versus $1,821 for people in the regular hospital.

- Miscellaneous other costs amounted to $278 in the palliative care unit and $2,152 for regular patients.

- The costs were closer for rooms and nursing, $3,708 in the palliative unit and $4,330 elsewhere, reflecting the human contact needs that rank highly in competent end-of-life care.

The five-day total: in the palliative care unit, $5,313; in the regular hospital, $12,319.

The difference was not due to scrimping on care. When a patient is no longer pursuing an unattainable cure, treatment is no longer dependent on the results of labs and imaging tests.

Remember, too, that the original goal was not to save money but to provide better care. It just turns out that in Richmond, better end-of-life treatment costs less than half what the current approach does.

IT WILL TAKE DECADES for hospitals to embrace the tenets of palliative care and thereby realize the potential savings. Quite possibly they will only do so when the population of elderly people grows so large that the current approach becomes unaffordable. In the meantime, health consumers could have a more immediate impact, through the use of advance directives.

These documents—which are legally binding but do not require a lawyer to produce—decree what values and priorities will determine a patient's care should he or she become unable to speak or make medical decisions.

Studies have found that patients who sign advance directives significantly lower the cost of their final hospitalization. Other research has determined that many of the potential economic gains of advance directives are missed because doctors and nurses either do not know the instructions are in place or ignore them. Still, one 1994 study estimated that if every patient who died in a previous year had written an advance directive, used hospice, and refused heroic intervention, it would have saved $18.1 billion—3.3 percent of all U.S health-care spending that year.

There is an immediate danger with findings like these. Economics offer arguably the weakest reason to reform end-of-life care. In fact, were money to lead the way in the discussion, the public would become understandably skeptical of reformers' motives. Suspicious that they are being directed to hospice only to save money, to die at home quietly and inexpensively, people could grow reluctant to embrace methods and a philosophy that actually promises to serve them well. They might perceive hospice as a form of rationing, one more brutal example of the abandonment of people who are dying.

This book's final chapter addresses in detail questions of how to encourage hospice and palliative care, and thereby realize potential savings, without triggering skepticism. For now, suffice it to say that the approach to care that provides greater comfort and dignity to patients also has the potential to reduce health-care expenditures.

That is good news for taxpayers. It is better news for families.

ONE IMPORTANT DIMENSION of families' woes does not appear in tallies of dollars and cents. But its emotional price can be far higher than is necessary or justified. It is the hidden cost of grief.

There is a time after a person has died, a few weeks or so, during which many families want the doctor to express a little sympathy, offer support, perhaps provide a time when they can ask questions. All evidence indicates that these legitimate expectations are rarely met.

Think of it: Friends and relatives of the person who died are struggling to make sense of one of the most emotional experiences in their lives, yet they do not even have a chance to ask, "What happened?"

That lost opportunity for clarity and healing is one simple indicator of how the medical system does not help families, because it cannot see beyond the person in the hospital bed: All contact dies with the patient.

This lost opportunity is due in part to a lack of time, which nearly every physician must reckon with. Partly it is due to a lack of empathy, as doctors turn away from the strong emotions of grieving people. The net result, though, is that well-intentioned healers can make the pain worse.

Researchers in the palliative care unit at Massachusetts General Hospital in Boston heard about this problem firsthand. In 1999 they surveyed relatives of people who had died in a nontraumatic way at that hospital over a three-month period. They found "an array of disturbing problems."

First, the people surveyed filled out a form, scoring their loved one's care on a scale of 0 to 5. The results were encouraging, averaging above 4 and showing a general satisfaction. But then the researchers interviewed the participants, who revealed "bitter criticisms and regrets."

Nearly 40 percent said they experienced a lack of respect. One woman was standing in a hallway when the doctor announced that her husband had died during surgery. "Why couldn't he have taken us to a private room?" Another widow said she had been rushed out of the room when her husband died. "I would have liked to have held him, to snuggle with him a little longer."

Communication problems were common, too. Relatives said, "When a family wants to talk with the doctor, they should be allowed to." One family reported arriving to find a loved one dead in his bed, and no one available who could say how he had died or when. Patients' advance directives were often ignored. So were simple requests to protect family members from unnecessary sorrow: "We told the hospital not to call my father because he couldn't take it, but when my mother died, they called him anyway."

Over a third of the family members reported no contact from the doctor after the patient died. Of those cases in which contact did occur, many times it was initiated by the family. The lingering bitterness was fierce: "After taking care of my dad for fourteen years, [the doctor] never called. I saw him in the street and crossed to the other side so I didn't have to face him." One family sent flowers to the hospital unit in gratitude but received no acknowledgment.

Perhaps worst was the mother who donated her twenty-five-year-old daughter's organs. "Doctors came from all over the country to get her body parts. I first thought it was a great idea. Then it occurred to me, they're chopping up my daughter. There was no follow-up. If they want more parents to give away their child, her actual being, how she smelled, how she felt, they must get someone to help the parents. I don't know where she is. I had nothing left to bury. It was a bigger sacrifice than I ever thought it would be."

Set aside for a moment how chilling this description is; there are compelling medical reasons for doctors and hospitals to pay attention to family members. First, organ donation is extremely important, with tens of thousands of Americans on waiting lists for transplants to aid their sight, free them from dialysis, and more. The emotions of donor families could inspire others to give, or could have the opposite effect.

Second, the death of a loved one affects the health of the family members. A woman whose child dies is four times as likely to die herself in the next three years. Simple bereavement services could lower the risk of these problems and identify those that occur before they become severe. One study of 35,000 couples found widows and widowers less likely to die within eighteen months of their spouse if their loved one received good end-of-life care.

Some people in the Mass General research sought bereavement assistance on their own; of the entire study group, though, only one person received a counseling referral from a doctor or nurse. Families scarcely mentioned the hospital's social workers and chaplains.

"Repeated, sustained bereavement support was lacking for all families," the study reports. As one participant simply stated, "I would have appreciated someone calling us to see how we were doing."

Three things are striking about the complaints of these grieving relatives. First, they are uniformly humble. Families are not demanding huge new services or extraordinary measures. They would like a sympathy note or a moment to talk to the doctor. Second, they are reasonable requests. No one should have to learn of a loved one's death while standing in a corridor. No one who donates a child's organs should feel so excluded that she comes to regret her generosity.

Third and most unfortunately, these complaints are all sad. The woman who did not get to hug her husband long enough will never have another chance. The family that wanted to protect its father from hearing bad news instead had to help him cope with it.

Humble, reasonable, and sad. Those are the dimensions of families' needs now that dying has become gradual. For all the wonders of health and longevity that modern medicine has wrought, these are the side effects—unintended and untreated. The wounds may never heal.

CHAPTER TWENTY-ONE

THE MOST IMPORTANT TIME

A baby is born into a community. The expectant mother attends birthing instruction, often with the father, and the room is filled with big-bellied women who share stories and excitement. Friends throw a baby shower to celebrate the imminent birth. When the child is born, grandparents visit, as do neighbors bearing food. Mothers bond at the playground and the pediatrician's office. Fathers find compatriots thanks to an infant strapped to their chest or riding in a backpack. Some of society's most embracing actions come in the community that forms around a new person.

The entrance to life could not be more different from the exit. People spend their final days in hospitals or nursing homes, often with little more companionship than a TV. As they become sicker, friends back away and doctors abandon them. Too often life's end is also its loneliest phase.

Imagine if the circumstances were different. Imagine if a person in the process of leaving this world remained in a community until his or her final breath.

Imagine if the health system helped families, saw them as people needing care, too, understood and valued their role. Imagine the power of a partnership between families and health-care professionals. Doctors and nurses have medical expertise but do not know the patients or their values. Families have the love and the sense of impending loss jointly motivating them to provide tender loving care, but do not know what medical choices will maximize a patient's quality of life.

Imagine if the professionals and the families joined forces and found support in the surrounding community. Together they could accomplish something every bit as sweet as the welcoming of an infant. Together they could make possible a final chapter as immersed in loving community as that of Betty Goyette.

BETTY BRAULT WAS BORN IN WINOOSKI, a tiny city clustered around defunct woolen mills in northwestern Vermont. She was the daughter of a barber. When she was a nursing student in the early 1950s, Betty went to a mixer at St. Michael's College. There she met Arthur Goyette, a mustachioed student from across the river in Burlington.

They married in 1958 and produced five children: Cathy, Anne, Michael, Susan, and David. Betty left nursing to raise the family. Art joined his father's wholesaling business. They bought a home in a neighborhood known as the Five Sisters, because the streets had girls' names. Living on Caroline Street, the children had a short walk to school and to the park. Betty needed only a minute to get to Christ the King Church, where she directed the choir. Although Betty never had time or money for voice lessons, every December 24 midnight Mass she would sing "O Holy Night" as a solo. In that church her performance was almost as much a part of the season as Santa.

Betty and Art, neighbors say, made a cute couple. They were busy but kept their romance strong with long walks in all weather. They would make the rounds of the Five Sisters at noontime or stroll down to Lake Champlain for the sunset. Nearly always they returned holding hands.

Art and Betty were surrounded by people raising young families. Yet the tradition of long walks continued over decades, as children went to college, married, moved across the country, formed families of their own.

In April 1998 doctors found that Betty had an ovarian tumor. The family instantly opted to use the full horsepower of medical intervention.

"The operation to take it out was supposed to take three hours," Art says. "It turned out seven."

The tumor weighed ten pounds. Betty underwent chemotherapy, in case the cancer was elsewhere in her body, and radiation to scour the tumor site. It was a grueling six months. When the treatment ended, the family celebrated.

"We went up to the hospital, and we brought champagne," recalls Betty's daughter Susan Brodeur. "We had a huge poster board, with pictures of men at the top of a mountain, and the words 'You did it!'"

Even then, the family realized that their approach was unusual.

"We saw lots of people going into chemo by themselves. They had the turbans on their heads, you know? That was how you knew why they were there. They were alone. And you felt sad, because you could see that there are a lot of those people."

The aggressive measures worked, and Betty had a series of checkups at which she received a clean bill of health. On the one-year anniversary of Betty being cancer-free, the family threw another party. Ovarian cancer is notoriously persistent, but Betty was, her family hoped and believed, cured.

In 2001 doctors found a new tumor. This time it was in Betty's brain. She had another operation, right away. Afterward her short-term memory was compromised, her balance unsteady. She healed more slowly and required more care. Art loved the caretaking, though, the quiet intimacy of it.

Ten months later Betty had another brain tumor. "It was the same cancer, in the same place," Art says. "Again she elected to have the surgery. I couldn't believe she'd do it a second time."

But she had a powerful will to live. Also, Art recalls, she completely trusted her doctor. Betty's recovery from that operation was the toughest yet. So was Art's role. "I called it a thirty-six-hours-a-day job," Art says. "Hey, the washer's in the cellar, the bedroom's upstairs."

Again the family put on an optimistic face and celebrated Betty's birthday. "After all her surgeries, she was not totally there in terms of being one hundred percent," Susan says. "But I gave her a magic wand. She was waving it over her cake, just being my mom, the silly, crazy lady she always was. It's hard to put into words, but there were so many moments that were really just about living."

That Christmas Eve, as usual, Betty was slated to sing "O Holy Night." At the service, though, she had an unbearable headache. Her son David ran home and brought back painkillers, and she went on with the song. Susan, on a whim, recorded the performance.

In April of 2002, now four years after her initial diagnosis, Betty started having trouble turning her head. One of her eyes began closing involuntarily as well. This time doctors found a tumor in her neck. It was large enough that Art could feel it with his fingers.

Still her determination was firm. Offered a chance to join an experimental chemotherapy trial, Betty said yes at once. Her physician said whoa, Art recalls. "You need to meet with the people, the doctors, and hear what it's about."

She moved ahead anyway. Under the treatment, within days Art could not feel the tumor anymore. "In two weeks the eye started opening up."

Up to this point, Betty's experience embodied the recent progress in cancer treatment. That is, two decades earlier she would simply have died, another of ovarian cancer's many victims. Instead, she lived additional years, with a wealth of experiences.

Unlike most people, however, Betty's next eighteen months defied the pattern of Americans dying slowly. Her will to live, her family's determination, her medical providers' excellent care, and her community's support created an experience well outside the norm.

The immediate pressures did not fall on her, though, but on Art. Maintaining Betty's dignity was a formidable task.

"She was in a wheelchair, and I didn't want to strap her in," he remembers. "But you need to do the dishes, or the phone rings and you turn your head for a second. Then she'd see a bit of dust, forget that she was in the chair, and reach for it without thinking. And, bang, down."

Art kept a tally: Betty fell sixty-one times. He frowns at the memory. "I ended up using the belt, bedrails, monitors."

As she had been weakened by so many surgeries and rounds of chemotherapy, Betty's needs grew. She became incontinent, so Art started getting up with her several times a night. His gratification from caretaking more than compensated for embarrassment or lost sleep. "It was a labor of love," he says. "I'd do it again in a heartbeat."

The work paid a priceless wage, too. Betty and Art celebrated their fortieth wedding anniversary, forty-first, forty-second. Their eldest daughter had a second child. They escaped winter by visiting their son Michael in Arizona. That summer Art bought Betty the singing lessons she'd always wanted. She practiced in her wheelchair or lying in bed.

One side effect of Betty's fight, however, was that it aged Art. Her nearly constant needs meant he had to wake up during the night just to do laundry and pay the bills. Their children became concerned for his health.

"By late November 2002 we could see more and more frustration happening with my father," Susan remembers. "It was no fault of his. He was getting up every two hours to make sure Mom was dry. That November we took a trip to visit my sister in San Diego. My dad was sort of at the breaking point. He was extremely exhausted, and much more having my sister and I fill in. In a tense situation he said, 'I can't do this anymore.' He said it in front of my mom, too. We didn't want her to feel like a burden. And he didn't mean it. He was just mentally and physically exhausted. I had been visiting them at home all along, but those were brief. On that trip I spent day in and day out with him, and that changed my perspective."

They returned home to the same demanding routine. Eventually, because the long Vermont winter shows no mercy to those who are not getting enough sleep, Art became ill.

"Pneumonia," he says. "I had stopped taking care of myself, and it caught up with me."

All the stair climbing aggravated an old knee injury as well. In April Art had arthroscopic surgery. His mobility was limited for a few weeks.

At that point, however, something unique began to happen. Betty's illness started to involve not just her family but the surrounding community. Residents of the Five Sisters area pitched in. They brought meal upon meal. They helped with household tasks. One neighbor began taking the Goyettes' garbage to the dump.

"You might think that's an odd chore to take on," Art says, "but it was a huge help. One less thing for me to do, so I could take care of Betty."

One spring day when a neighbor was dropping off a casserole, Art happened to mention that Betty had never ridden in a convertible. "A few days later the doorbell rings, and there's a Chrysler Sebring convertible, brand-new, like about six thousand miles on it," Art recalls. "It wasn't perfect weather, but we had a great ride. Betty was in there like a queen, neighbors taking pictures. We went and got the grandkids and took them for a creemie.

"Two days later the woman rings again. She says the weather wasn't so great last time, and here's another Sebring."

While these efforts lifted Art's morale, his stamina was flagging. "It was too much, and I resisted getting help. But I couldn't do a thing, write a check or anything. So I'd get up early in the morning, turn on the monitor, and get busy. When she woke up, I'd run up the stairs."

A friend told Art about hospice, to help with nursing, provide aides for nonmedical tasks like bathing, and bring volunteers to visit with Betty. The message didn't sink in.

During one of Betty's appointments with her oncologist, Art received a brochure about hospice. It was in a stack of informational materials, and he set them all aside.

"He didn't want to give up that ownership of her care," Susan says. "He knew her medications schedule. He had timers going off 24/7. That man never missed a beat with her."

For her part, Betty began making decisions. No more interventions. No more extreme measures. The cancer was not gone, Art says, but her interest in tracking its spread was. "Why spend six hundred dollars for a CAT scan when she doesn't want any more surgery or chemo?" Art asks.

Amid the growing strain, Susan ran into an old friend with whom she'd been involved in a youth charity. The friend's sister had died in the care of the local hospice organization. In her final days the sister had lived in the Vermont Respite House, a fourteen-bed residential facility in nearby Williston. The house was available for people in the hospice program who for whatever reason could not remain in their homes.

"I only knew that the Respite House was a place you went to die," Susan says. But her friend was enthusiastic about the quality of care and the attention to patient dignity.

Susan called the local nonprofit that provides home health care and hospice services and runs Respite House.

"The woman in charge asked if my mother was still receiving chemotherapy or radiation treatment," Susan says. If she were, Betty would have been ineligible; Medicare pays for hospice only if people have ceased curative treatment. Betty fit the criteria.

"Next she said they would interview the family and see whether we were ready for hospice care in the home," Susan says. "And a social worker would talk to my mother, to see if she was ready, too."

It was encouraging news, because Art might receive some help. But it was awkward as well. The severity of Betty's illness and the strain on Art would be out in the open. Susan dealt with the situation by waiting to call back to schedule the visits until she was at her parents' house. In the middle of the conversation, she handed her father the phone.

Art spoke softly, introducing himself and listening to the woman on the other end. All at once the message of help came through at last.

"I was bawling on the phone, and the woman was telling us that we were definitely eligible," he remembers. "One thing I'll never forget: The woman's name was Angel."

ANGEL COLLINS is a former respiratory therapist who specialized in ventilator care for terminal patients, "for years at a time, sometimes."

After ten years in the field, Angel began to question whether patients were well served by medical aggressiveness. "I remember being involved in one code blue after another, and we had no idea what their wishes were," she recalled. "We just cracked the chest, and then only after wondered, 'My God, what have I done?' Nobody ever presented the alternatives."

Angel's specialty also meant that she often performed the task of disconnecting a person from ventilator support—a step that typically invites death to come within minutes or hours. One day while removing a patient's breathing tube, she realized they were the only people in the room.

"There was no one there for the person in the bed," she said. "There was no respect for family members. There was no thought of the effect on the caregiver. It was a huge awakening."

Angel quit that job and went to nursing school. She focused on learning to provide dignified end-of-life care to cancer patients. In addition to its emotional rewards, the shift was good for her career. Today she is associate director of hospice for the Visiting Nurse Association of Chittenden and Grand Isle Counties—a home health company serving the 170,000 people in Art's corner of Vermont.

"There is a privilege in this work that we all feel, understanding the humanity of our patients," Angel said. "There is a window they open for us that they don't open for others and can't address in a thirty-minute meeting in a physician's office.

"As a society we are slowly, slowly moving from seeing death as failure to accepting death as a normal and natural part of life.

"What if, as a culture, people could trust that they would be heard, that there is no shame, that they would be cared for at the very last moment? If we do our job right, people may die more content and fulfilled than they ever were back in their healthy days. That is why we say that while we may not cure, we do accomplish healing."

Soon a nurse arrived to help with Betty's medical needs. An aide began coming three times a week to bathe her. Hospice volunteers showed up to help Art with household tasks. They also kept Betty company while he did errands, shopped for groceries, or took a moment to catch his breath.

"It was a process for my father to relinquish the day-to-day purpose of his taking care of mom," Susan says. "Handing it over to people he didn't know, he had to rely on faith. He had to trust these people."

Art's feelings of relief came quickly. He was struck by the volunteers' level of commitment to a stranger. "They have all become friends," he says. "They certainly were friends to Betty, every one of them."

The hospice in Art's county has 225 volunteers, Angel said. "It is a fundamental component of the hospice mission to involve the community."

166 · LAST RIGHTS

It is also a requirement. Medicare reimburses a health organization for hospice care only if volunteers participate. The purpose is plain: Volunteers prove that caring for people who are dying is not the sole province of health professionals; it must involve the community.

Few hospices suffer for a lack of volunteers, though. People whose loved ones have died in the bosom of hospice care frequently become volunteers, financial donors, and advocates. Their support provides tangible evidence of the quality of care their loved ones received.

After a few weeks the family prepared to move Betty to the Respite House. Situated in a neighborhood that borders a small-scale commercial area, the facility looks nothing like a hospital. There are picnic tables, gardens, bird feeders outside each room's windows.

Art asked Susan to do the packing. "He had enough on his plate," she says. Susan chose pictures of her parents' wedding, photos of close friends, a stuffed animal she'd given her mother before the first surgery. Susan's husband brought flowers to Betty's room.

Even so, the transition was confusing for Betty. "She was scared," Susan says. "At first my mom thought it was just a temporary thing. 'I'm just here, right, until Dad gets better?' I don't know how cognizant she was."

However, Betty soon settled in. The family added decorations almost daily, photos and cards. Susan ran a marathon wearing a T-shirt on which she'd written "Miles for Mom"; the shirt wound up on the wall.

With friends visiting, volunteers coming regularly, and Art regaining his health, Betty began to feel more at home. In May the Respite House held a fund-raising 5K road race. Susan ran in it, and most of the family came for the event. Afterward they gathered for a photo, Betty in her wig and a wide straw hat, Art behind her wheelchair like a bodyguard. It was a sunny day, with music and prizes and three hundred runners. A sweaty stranger squatted beside Betty's chair and asked if she was having a good day.

She smiled. "Every day is a good day."

By midsummer Betty's condition had taken a downward turn. She was less responsive. She needed more pain medication. She slept more. Volunteers would spend the morning with Betty, then Art would come, leaving only after she had gone to sleep at night.

Driving home alone and arriving at an empty house, Art used these routines to prepare for the future. One day there would be a last drive back to Caroline Street from the Respite House.

Meanwhile, Art reconnected with friends and replenished his strength for the task that lay ahead. A perennial duffer, he even began sporadically playing golf again. That presented an opportunity for Betty to show that her sense of humor remained intact.

One day he shot his lowest score ever, a personal best. "I was bragging about it, and Betty had had enough, I guess. She said, 'Big deal.' Then she twirled her pinkie in the air and said, 'And put a pink ribbon on it.'

"We all roared," Art says.

Another day he asked Betty if she wanted a priest to hear her confession. She grinned at him and said, "I can't do anything in here, can I?"

As summer turned to fall, light moments became rare. Yet the weaker Betty became, the more her family showed a determination to help. For her sixty-sixth birthday, they threw yet another party. Susan dressed up as a clown. There were grandchildren, balloons, a cake. Members of the choir Betty had directed for decades came and sang to her.

The volunteers continued doing their part, too. One brought berries, which Betty loved. Another painted her toenails. "She is still getting her soul fed with this loving care from so many," Art says. "It's part of what keeps her alive."

The family members remained acutely aware of how lucky they were.

"Some of the other people at the Respite House, they didn't have a lot of visitors," Susan remembers. "It was sad. We found ourselves connecting with people at the dinner table, and later going down to visit them in their rooms."

The Respite House had a huge hand in the quality of Betty's life, constantly applying personalized hospice principles. Music played at her bedside. She had plants in her room. When Betty slept late one day, the cafeteria staffer said, "You don't want breakfast, you want brunch."

Medically, too, her care was exemplary. The staff worked to balance Betty's pain medications with her desire to be alert whenever possible. For example, when her nursing school held a reunion and a group of old classmates came to visit, she was bright and present.

Times were not always sweet, though; no medical model can eliminate loss. Betty's sisters brought her a new outfit, but they had to cut the back open to get it on her without causing too much pain. On Art's birthday he brought cards he'd received to the Respite House so he could open them with Betty. She did not understand. When he tried to explain, she became confused and agitated.

Yet Art's face brightens at the memory. "I guess they could tell I was feeling low about that, because at lunch all the Respite House folks came out banging pots and pans and singing me 'Happy Birthday.'"

As his knee healed, Art began taking walks again—but now he was alone. Often he went to the same place he'd gone with Betty so many times, down by Lake Champlain for the sunset. "Is it preparation?" he says. "Yes."

He let less urgent tasks go. He didn't finish his taxes till August 13. "Look at my lawn out front. Well, the lawn will be there after."

One Sunday the family gathered to write Betty's obituary. "Writing it was not as sorrowful as you'd think," Art says. "It was fun in a way. No, not fun. But it was really something to be writing down who she is."

Art had one thing he wanted to include in the obituary that had little to do with Betty. After what Medicare paid, the Respite House was costing him $170 a day. That was 20 percent less than even a mediocre nursing home but amounted to a considerable sum over the six months she lived at the facility. At the end of the obituary he added a request that, in lieu of flowers, contributions be made to the Respite House. "This way somebody else might enjoy what we all took from there," he said.

Few other details remained. Art purchased a plot in Resurrection Park Cemetery in South Burlington. He selected Betty's casket. "That wasn't as bad as I thought it would be. The guy was very nice. And I'm trying to do these things when you're not under the emotional strain of afterward."

"Afterward" became Art's euphemism for life after Betty, a time he deliberately did not give much contemplation. "I just wonder how it will be, when I don't have this fulfilling my life. I like to tell myself I'm okay. I still have some purpose in life."

After her third surgery, Betty had started collecting Mass cards, prayers, and hymns. Art kept the thick file on the dining-room table and flipped through papers matter-of-factly. "There are lots of good ideas in here." He stopped at one card, a list of songs. "She picked the ones for her funeral, of course. A choir director will do that."

He pointed at her selection for the offertory hymn: "Be Not Afraid."

A FEW DAYS LATER Art and Betty were sitting in the Respite House's dining room when an old song they'd loved came on the radio. Betty's face took on a poignant expression. Art stood behind her wheelchair and guided her in small circles around the room. It was the closest they would come to having a last dance.

At about that time Betty's hands began to swell, and a jeweler had to remove her wedding ring. A childhood friend had given Betty a hot-pink scarf to wear whenever her wig became uncomfortable. Art wrapped the scarf around Betty's shoulders, then threaded it through his ring before knotting it on her chest. "That way I could be with her all the time," Art says. Then he put her ring on a necklace, which he wears to this day.

Such incidents made Art philosophical about the immediate future. "I am glad that she has fought as hard as she has. She has been an example to so many people. Her faith is strong for people, too, certainly to my kids.

"She is at peace now. She told me two nights ago that she wants to live, she's got so much going on, family and stuff. But she's ready. She's at peace. I am ready to let her go. I don't want to, but it's her battle. I have told her, 'I'll do anything you want to keep you going.' I also told her I am willing to let her go.

"She's certainly had enough. You have to say your good-byes and let them know it's all okay."

By late August Betty was sleeping almost all the time. Nearly five and a half years had passed since her first diagnosis. Her affairs were in order, she had often spent time with a priest, all was prepared.

There was one remaining difficulty: her son Michael refused to come from Arizona to see her. Art was disappointed, and Susan had written Michael a scathing letter, "trying to guilt him into coming home," she says.

The only person who did not seem agitated about it was Betty.

"That was how she kept mothering us, you see?" Susan says. "Still teaching us. She was not upset, because she knew her son best. She understood him and loved him for who he was. And that was what she wanted us to do, too."

Betty's appetite dwindled, and on September 12 it stopped altogether. Her thirst waned as well. On the twentieth Art arrived with a dozen roses for Betty to mark their forty-fifth wedding anniversary. He announced his intention of kissing her forty-five times to mark the occasion. He leaned over the bed and counted each time their lips touched. Though she had not spoken more than a few words at a time for three weeks, they looked directly into each other's eyes. About halfway through the kisses, one of their children asked Art a question.

"Well, now I've lost count," he said, never turning his face from Betty's. "I guess I'll have to start over."

And she smiled. Her hair was gone, her skin waxy, her personality less manifest with each hour. But in that moment of love and family and humor, Betty smiled.

Without food and water, Respite House workers told Art, Betty would live about ten more days. Slowly her life quieted. Friends visited. Her family drew close, said their good-byes, declared their love, stayed at the Respite House day and night. Sleep and the pain drugs took over. Betty's room became a place of silence and peace.

The afternoon of September 24 Betty's breathing grew labored. Two staffers stayed after their shift ended, thinking her time was close. Finally at midnight they agreed to Art's entreaties to go home, but only after making him promise that he would call if she died—no matter what time it was.

About 3:15 A.M., Art was lying with Betty in her bed as her breath came more and more slowly, with longer lapses in between. He held her in his arms. He prayed. He leaned over and kissed her on the lips.

"And that was it," he recalls. "Betty finished her journey."

ART KEPT HIS PROMISE and called the hospice workers at home. One of the women came immediately, stayed with the family, and cried with them. After a while she asked Art to leave Betty's room for a few minutes. Soon she invited him back in.

The room was lit by scented candles. The bed was neatly made. Betty wore fresh clothes and lipstick. There were family pictures on the bedside table. One of Betty's hands was folded around a rose, the other held her rosary. Around her neck the pink scarf was knotted neatly.

"Talk about a final gift," Art says. "She was relaxed, the fight was over, and she was so beautiful anyway. I watched the kids as they came in, and they all saw how beautiful she looked."

The Respite House gave the family all the time they wanted in Betty's room. They stayed till nearly dawn. Susan and David returned a few days later to remove all the decorations; it took hours. In keeping with the facility's policy, Betty's room remained vacant for several more days, occupied only by a lit candle, allowing the staff time to grieve and accept and become calm with her death.

The wake took place on a rainy September afternoon. The crowd was huge, eight hundred people waiting to pay their respects. Michael was there.

By then Susan had put his decision to stay away in a new perspective. "Cathy came home from San Diego monthly. Anne and David and I were here and visiting with her all the time, so we saw each step in Mom's illness. It was all gradual, and we got to absorb it on a daily basis. But Michael, he was in Arizona, and he only got to see her a few times, with a long time in between. For him, the changes were a disaster. Like one time he came home, and to see my mom in a wheelchair? We were used to it, but he didn't know what to do with her."

Michael knelt by his mother's casket and broke down crying. Susan knelt beside him.

"He was saying, 'I'm sorry, I'm sorry.' Then he said, 'Do you think she's angry at me?' I told him, 'No. She was at peace. It wasn't about whether you were here or not. She loved you unconditionally.'"

Susan rates that conversation as one of the most important and meaningful of her life.

Betty's funeral took place at the neighborhood church, where she'd been hundreds of times. When the procession began, Art started down the aisle, then glanced back. "There's my oldest daughter with her arms spread around all the kids, they're all hugging. We've always been close, but this experience just unified the family."

During the offertory, while the organist played "Be Not Afraid," two of Betty's children brought forward the gifts—the bread, the wine, and one hot-pink scarf.

After the Mass, the songs sung by children and grandchildren and the eulogy delivered by David, Betty's family turned on a tape player. It was a fuzzy recording, the organ music difficult at first to decipher. Then a clear, strong soprano began singing "O Holy Night."

The church went completely quiet. Still, after half a minute, David went forward and turned the player up loud. While people in the congregation wept, Betty's family stood beaming.

After the song ended, Art leaned forward and snatched the scarf off the casket. "I didn't want to be too flamboyant. I was putting it in my pocket when my daughter pulled it out and said, 'You should wear that.'"

Art draped the scarf over his shoulder, a bright flag against his dark suit. "The hell with what people thought. It was her funeral, our celebration. I wore it with my head up."

The scarf remained on Art's shoulder during the committal at the cemetery, at the social gathering afterward, and for the rest of the day.

THERE ARE TWO IMMEDIATE DANGERS in a story like the Goyettes'.

The first is the temptation to dismiss their case as something special. True, their experience defies the statistics about people dying in pain, feeling abandoned, and receiving unwanted medical interventions. True, too, their family was unusually loving and free of dysfunction. But these were not people of any otherwise special circumstances. They did not have advanced degrees. They did not work in health care. They were not political activists or social advocates or participants in any other form of engagement with society that would make them more assertive in medical demands. They were not wealthy. They were not zealots.

What, then, distinguishes Betty's care? Her family's involvement and eventual openness to hospice played an important role. But the other crucial difference was that her medical care was consistently good. Betty managed to wrest five and a half years away from an aggressive ovarian cancer. She survived three surgeries, two of them on her brain. She underwent two rounds of chemotherapy, one of them an experiment that by many measures worked well. She received radiation around her original tumor site, which evidently succeeded, since the disease never recurred in that place. Her pain was controlled with a keen eye toward balancing alertness with relief.

Her care was also expertly managed. Betty's doctor hesitated before embarking on the chemotherapy trial, a sign that even in the experiment she remained more a person than a statistic. The strategy for her care evolved as her illness did. Art received numerous suggestions to explore hospice. Once Betty entered that system, she was treated as an individual and her whole family received care. Art participated in a support group for families of people in hospice before she died, for example, and received bereavement services afterward.

Perhaps the clearest indicator of the quality of Betty's treatment is that the first phone call Art received on the morning after she died—the very first one—was a call of condolence from her oncologist. So simple, so appropriate, so rare.

This is why Betty's story cannot be shrugged off as one family's good luck. It was actually the result of many systems working as correctly for her as they should for all people nearing death.

BY CONTRAST, for the majority of people in situations like Betty's, the care is simply not good enough.

One authoritative study of family members' perceptions found that "severe fatigue affected almost 8 in 10 patients. . . . Sixty-three percent of patients had difficulty tolerating physical or emotional symptoms.

"In addition, 17 percent of family members reported that patients felt alone and isolated the last three days of life. More than one in three conscious patients had severe pain, even in disease categories in which severe pain might not have been expected. Almost 70 percent of conscious patients who died with lung cancer or multiple organ failure with a malignant condition had severe" problems with shortness of breath.

Consequently, one sure way doctors and administrators could reduce conflicts with families would be to improve the quality of care. When patients are not in pain and are not suffering needlessly from their symptoms, families have far less reason to stand in a doctor's way.

The *Annals of Internal Medicine* article reporting that doctors regard families as the primary source of trouble suggests that care providers adopt a more compassionate perspective:

> *A system that saves or prolongs lives only to cast patients and families into the abyss of fragmented chronic care and financial and emotional ruin, while at the same time criticizing them for being "too emotional," is unjust. Many families are willing to make enormous sacrifices, but martyrdom is not a good basis for health care policy or practice. . . . A health care system that depends so heavily on the patient care and management provided by families should involve families as partners rather than define them as problems.*

Exactly.

THERE IS A SECOND DANGER to the Goyettes' story, and it lies in their nearly ideal behavior during trying circumstances.

The point does not bear dwelling on in depth, but it is obviously true that not every family member acts out of total, loving, selfless generosity. Sometimes people behave based on old hurts. Sometimes people distrust authority figures like doctors without basis. Sometimes people are incapable of putting themselves anywhere but at the top of the list of family priorities. Some people find fulfillment in playing the martyr or in manipulating others or in making sure everyone knows how inconvenient and distressing their loved one's dying is for them.

Likewise, some doctors are petty or easily annoyed by the people they treat. Some see a diagnosis instead of a person. Some cannot silence the clock in their head—urging them on to the next appointment or meeting—long enough to be fully present with the patient and family at hand. Some doctors misconstrue families' deference as a sign of their own power and importance. Some, full of their training and status and income, condescend.

Unfortunately, there is no cure for human nature. Fallibility is with us always; it only manifests itself with greater clarity in the harsh lighting that can surround a person nearing the end of his or her life.

Ironically, patients can exacerbate these problems. Because they are accustomed to a leading role in the family, for example, parents can have huge attachment to their dignity and authority. Dependency—physical, emotional, or financial—can be harder for them to swallow than any medicine.

That challenge, and the many others that patients face in their final journeys, is the subject of the next chapter. While some of those obstacles are formidable, many people have accomplished inspirational ends to their lives—their relationships strong and preparations made, and all manner of last wishes fulfilled. When people die with dignity, they leave behind loved ones at peace.

And when a family contributes to a physically comfortable and emotionally supportive dying experience, it creates something entirely new. Yes, the family members will feel loss. But as that grief abates, over time they experience another set of emotions, all positive: one part relief for themselves and the one who died, one part gratification at doing a hard task well, and three parts pride because of what they accomplished by turning a loved one's last chapter into a time of closeness and compassion and care. As this new kind of dying takes hold in contemporary America, these few fortunate families are discovering a new kind of love.

Art Goyette knows. Two months after Betty's death, he went to a forum on end-of-life care that included a debate about legalizing physician-assisted suicide. After sitting quietly for two hours, he stood.

"People are cheating themselves" if they hasten the death of a loved one, Art said. "They are robbing themselves of probably the most meaningful time in their life."

After the forum Art spoke easily of Betty's death. "People say, 'You must be so sad.' But I tell them no. I feel great. It was the most beautiful process of my life.

"I had forty-five good years of marriage. I had three years of courting before that. And I was allowed the privilege of kissing her right before she died. Anything more than that, I would be getting greedy."

The Respite House received hundreds of donations in Betty's name, thousands of dollars. Art penned a thank-you note to every person. He also wrote to his children, "telling them that I have never been so proud of them, and how much I have drawn strength from them."

Months later a local cancer survivors' organization was holding a fund-raising walk and invited Art to speak. He titled his remarks "The Most Important Time in Your Life."

Art drove around New England with David, revisiting places he'd traveled with Betty. He flew to Arizona to see Michael, and to California to visit Cathy. He plays golf and takes long walks timed to capture lakeside sunsets. The six months Betty lived at the Respite House prepared him for being alone, he says. "That's been a huge help in adjusting."

Beyond family, his purpose is an unknown, Art says. "I haven't gone back to any organizations I was involved in. . . . I think I want some new experiences. I am definitely taking my time."

Meanwhile, every night Art walks up the stairs of the house he and Betty shared for more than forty years and climbs into bed. There, knotted on the bedpost on Betty's side, hangs a bright pink scarf.

PART FIVE

SMELLING THE ROSES

Fear no more the heat o' the sun,
Nor the furious winter's rages;
Thou thy worldly task hast done,
Home art gone, and ta'en thy wages:
Golden lads and girls all must,
As chimney-sweepers, come to dust.

Fear no more the frown o' the great,
Thou art past the tyrant's stroke;
Care no more to clothe and eat;
To thee the reed is as the oak:
The sceptre, learning, physic, must
All follow this, and come to dust.

—WILLIAM SHAKESPEARE

CHAPTER TWENTY-TWO

"HER WISHES WERE TOTALLY IGNORED"

Katherine Kemp Cross of Palm Beach, Florida, took her first breaths in the rarefied atmosphere of privilege. She was born the daughter of a successful Toronto industrialist who had significant holdings in steel. How significant? During World War I, when the Canadian government was struggling to fund its military, her father stepped in. He wrote personal checks to underwrite the war effort. The checks were not only large enough to make a difference, they also caused the king of England to be grateful. After the war he knighted Katherine's father, making him Sir Edward Kemp.

Those were Katherine's beginnings, and they endured. She met a Yale man, the scion of a Pennsylvania brick-manufacturing empire. In 1954 they married, moved to a tony suburb of Pittsburgh, and before long had three children. Katherine was famously attractive. When the upscale magazine *Town & Country* published a feature on the lives of the well-heeled in Pittsburgh, Katherine warranted her own page of photographs.

Over the years the marriage soured, and she divorced in 1964. Katherine moved to Florida, and a few years later married James Cross—another Yale alumnus. It was a long, happy relationship, until he died in 1998.

Shortly beforehand James confided in Katherine's daughter Dana.

"He said she had a lump in her breast," Dana said. "She refused to talk about it, though, or to do anything about it. But he thought I ought to know. It was a terrible predicament, because he had unburdened himself, but I wasn't supposed to even bring it up in front of her."

Katherine was unwell in other ways, too. She had suffered bouts of depression, and after James died her condition worsened dramatically. She became lethargic, let social connections lapse, grew increasingly isolated and downhearted. From her lofty beginnings, it was a long way down. "At the end she had no friends at all," Dana said.

In 2000 Katherine finally confessed to Dana that she had breast cancer. The tumor was the size of a fist. Then Katherine's housekeeper, in her broken English, shared another secret: Sometimes she had to wash the sheets because they were stained with blood.

Katherine refused all treatment for her condition, year upon year. No surgery, no chemotherapy. "I think she hoped it would just get her," Dana said. "She wanted to be relieved of her painful existence."

Ironically, the cancer never spread. Katherine lived on. Meanwhile, though, her mental illness worsened. She developed psychotic dementia, periodically losing touch with reality. While not dangerous, Katherine's illusions were vivid and strange.

"I was visiting her and went out one night," Dana remembered. "When I came back there was a note to the houseguests to let the dog in when they came home. But there were no houseguests. There was no dog.

"Another time she told me she'd just been on a cruise with her sister on the QE2. Of course, her sister had been dead for over twenty years."

Even in lucid times, Katherine suffered. "It was so bad," Dana said. "She was just intensely unhappy. She had been a real knockout. But when she went down? Whoa."

During one of her cogent periods, Katherine drew up advance directives: no resuscitation, no ventilators, no feeding tubes, no dialysis. She sent copies to Dana, her son in Ohio, and her daughter in Pennsylvania. Katherine even underlined important parts in pink pen.

"I remember seeing the language," Dana said. "'Do not stick tubes in me, do not take any extraordinary measures.' I thought, boy, that sounds like her. She didn't want to risk anything keeping her alive."

One day in November 2001 the housekeeper found Katherine on the living-room floor and immediately called an ambulance.

Katherine told the EMTs that no one could force her to ride to the hospital, Dana said. "She refused to go. The medics said they would see how she was in twenty-four hours."

The next morning the housekeeper found Katherine in even worse condition. "She was not moving, completely unresponsive," Dana said. "She had nine toes in the grave. But the housekeeper called the ambulance again.

"They took her and completely intubated her, every tube, every single thing she didn't want. They plugged her into every single thing they could."

No one checked to see if there was an advance directive in place. Instead, the three children received a call that their mother had been hospitalized. With the idiosyncrasies of airline schedules, Dana could not get on a plane to Florida till late in the day. Her siblings caught earlier flights, and in a few hours Dana's sister called from Katherine's bedside.

"My mother was in a straitjacket in the bed, strapped down so she couldn't move," Dana said. "She was trying to rip it out, anything she could. She was writhing, my sister used that word on the phone with me, writhing in misery."

A little while later Dana had her chance to say good-bye as her sister held the phone to Katherine's ear. Dana was sitting at her desk in an open office. She spoke her heart anyway. Her mother did not respond.

"She was way gone by then. But while I was talking to her, my brother told me, they could see her blood pressure rise."

The family told the medical team to remove Katherine's life support. Dana's sister recounted that process over the phone, too.

"The morphine started before they disconnected. I asked my sister, 'Did you see the crease in her forehead?' She said yes, but every time it raised they'd give her more morphine, until she just drifted off."

It was November 21, 2001. On her flight to Florida that evening, Dana felt a mix of emotions: grief that her mother was gone, relief that her suffering was over, and something else, too—an emotion that remains strong even now. Rage.

"When I think of my mother in a straitjacket so she couldn't pull out her tubes like she was trying to do, it really angers me."

Dana arrived late that night. In the morning she went to the funeral home. "This was going to be the first dead person I had ever seen. It's a little freaky."

When she was led to her mother's body, though, "I didn't recognize her. I had expected to see someone who was gray and pale, sure. But I also expected to see her face. I mean, she hadn't been gone very long. But all the tubes they'd shoved in her mouth had completely distorted her features. It wasn't her face. It was so bad, the funeral home couldn't get her features all put back together."

She knew that her mother, despite the years of emotional hardship, had always been proud of her beautiful hands. Dana lifted up the sheet. "At least they looked normal. Her hands were still her hands, thank God."

Years later Dana remains angry about how worthless her mother's directives proved to be. "We all knew she wanted to go. We wanted her to be curled in her bed the way she wanted. Her wishes were totally ignored.

"It just shouldn't have been that way, damn it all."

CHAPTER TWENTY-THREE

THE DESIRE FOR CONTROL

Most people do not approach their final years battling the solitude and depression that Katherine faced. They want to live, and they want their quality of life to be as high as possible for as long as possible. But as a growing number of Americans watch their demise approaching slowly, they experience a desire very much like Katherine's: to be in control.

There is no cheating mortality, of course. But incremental dying presents many opportunities for people to control the shape of their final weeks, days, and hours. Just as the health-care system has been slow to evolve to accommodate the shift in dying, it has failed to honor the priorities—and some would say the rights—of patients who are still very much alive.

Consider, as a starting point, the advance directive Katherine put in place. Medical institutions have not exactly encouraged this simple step in patient empowerment. Depending on which research you read, between 5 and 30 percent of Americans have drafted these documents.

Advance directives typically take two forms. The first kind specifies the care people want to receive if they are unable to speak or otherwise express their wishes. The second kind gives the power to make medical decisions to another person, a proxy, some trusted relative or friend.

The simple existence of these documents proves that there are options in the last phase of life, decisions that can alter its course and meaning. Moreover, the reasonable premise is that during gradual dying, physicians—for all their clinical expertise—serve less of a central role and more of a consulting function. Patients are in charge.

Or at least they want to be. The Institute of Medicine cites a Harris poll that found when people were asked who should make care choices should they become seriously ill, only 28 percent wanted their doctor to decide. Instead, 67 percent wanted to make the call themselves.

These numbers are not surprising, given shifting public attitudes. The culture has come a long way from physicians deciding, all by themselves, how much to tell patients about their condition. Consumer attitudes today are far less deferential. Autonomy and control are ever greater priorities, and not just in health care. More people are self-employed, more people handle their own investments, more people pump their own gas.

Earlier it was suggested that physician-assisted suicide offers the clearest consumer condemnation of the quality of American end-of-life care. But in Oregon, where assisted suicide is legal, it is interesting that the main reason most people exercise this option is not pain or suffering. Research shows that the primary motivation of people who initiate a physician-assisted suicide is the desire for control.

Historically the power of patients to determine their care, and especially to set limits on it, has not been a certainty. From a California Supreme Court case in 1960 up to the 2005 Justice Department challenge of Oregon's assisted-suicide law, courts have heard a long opera of arguments over whether people have a right to medical self-determination. The rulings in these cases have slowly reduced the paternalism inherent in traditional medicine, and now require doctors to treat people only when they have obtained their informed consent. That is, for major interventions, the patient must be aware of what is happening and what the risks and options are, and then must give permission before a doctor can act.

Other decisions have bolstered the power of surrogates to decide on behalf of a patient who cannot communicate. The 1976 Karen Ann Quinlan decision by the New Jersey Supreme Court permitted removal of her ventilator. The U.S. Supreme Court's 1990 ruling on Nancy Cruzan expanded the definition of life-prolonging treatments that may be removed to include feeding tubes. A 1991 case determined that doctors could not discontinue a patient's care, however futile, against her family's wishes. The prolonged Terry Schiavo case, resolved in Florida and federal courts in 2005, reaffirmed that spouses have the highest legal standing to make choices on behalf of patients who cannot speak for themselves.

These cases are culturally wrenching because decisions about end-of-life care are not suited to the glare of media attention or the clash of political interests. Rather, these choices are best made in quiet reflection, by people who are humbled by the potential consequences of their decisions. Still, the gradual effect of the legal tangles has been to strengthen the powers of patients and their surrogates to control the medical care of the terminally ill.

Congress also has attempted to help. The 1990 Patient Self-Determination Act requires health institutions that receive federal funds to provide adult patients with written information about advance directives. The law also prohibits discrimination against patients who have these instructions in place. Further, the act requires institutions to teach both their staff and the surrounding communities about advance directives.

Subsequent research has found many shortcomings with the law. Less than a third of the institutions performed the required community education. Meanwhile, patients typically received the information upon admission to the hospital or nursing home, amid a bundle of bureaucratic paper.

"The lack of involvement of physicians," the Institute of Medicine says, "contributes to the tendency of patients to overlook the information offered."

Still, some patients did fish the document out and prepare an advance directive. But when researchers looked, the medical charts of half of those people did not contain a copy.

That is miles shy of informing patients about possibly weighty decisions ahead. There is no Alzheimer's patient, for example, for whom questions about feeding tubes and antibiotics are moot. Many people with that form of dementia eventually stop eating, and many others contract pneumonia. A patient with either complication could decide to battle these problems, to prolong life, or could choose not to use these medical options, thus allowing death to occur at whatever pace nature dictates.

The challenge is that these complications arise in the disease's most advanced stage, when the patient lacks the cognitive clarity to weigh options, make decisions, and articulate what ought to be done. Planning ahead would enable the medical care to reflect the patient's desires. Would you want a feeding tube or not? Do you prefer to receive antibiotics or not?

This situation is not confined to Alzheimer's. Patients with emphysema are going to face questions about using a ventilator. Patients with end-stage lung disease are likely to have an intensive-care unit in their future—with feeding tubes, ventilator support, and, as the data resoundingly confirms, pain managed even less well than that of patients with cancer. Yet too often physicians do not initiate conversations about where these illnesses might lead and what provisions a patient might make just in case.

Think of it: The doctor is sitting there, in one office visit after another, knowing these problems are likely to occur but failing to raise them for discussion. Yet that is *precisely* the time when patients need to be engaged—not when the crisis arrives because they won't chew or can't breathe or need so much pain medicine that it will render them unconscious. At that point the caregivers and family must guess at the patients' desires, when the stakes could not possibly be higher. If family members cannot reach a consensus, then they become like any Americans who cannot agree on an important issue; they land in court. But no judge or jury or act of Congress is going to make these decisions an easy or automatic call.

It's a matter of addressing possible issues early, and of maintaining balance. The danger in giving patients complete control lies in their lack of seasoned medical judgment, for which there is no substitute. Ideally, the answer lies somewhere in the middle, whereby patients, families, and physicians cooperatively determine the best course—long before a crisis.

Because doctors don't initiate those conversations, medicine's least flattering traditions are alive and well. One study tracked doctors who received information on a terminal patient's prognosis and care preferences. Asked about it later, only about 60 percent of the physicians reported that they had the information. Only one-third even recalled receiving the information. In classic paternalistic fashion, they just weren't listening.

"The problem of physicians ignoring their patients' wishes goes beyond issues of communication," maintains an article in the *Annals of Internal Medicine*. Rather, it "reflects an ongoing ambivalence about power and control in the physician-patient relationship. Unfortunately, many physicians find it easier to define success in terms of life and death than to try to determine what sort of existence is meaningful to an individual patient."

Think back a moment to that doctor sitting in a room with a person who has Alzheimer's disease, yet has not raised the topics of feeding tubes and pneumonia care. Does the physician's silence reflect discomfort at broaching a sensitive subject, or something less conscious that has to do with control?

An editor of the *Journal of Palliative Medicine* framed this question for readers in personal terms. David Weissman, M.D., wrote an article about providing a palliative care consultation for an eighty-two-year-old man who had a kind of bone cancer called multiple myeloma, plus worsening pneumonia. Weissman met with the patient's family, reviewed the no-resuscitation, no-ventilator orders in place, and suggested medicines to manage pain and delirium. The next day he returned to find the patient much worse:

> As I came out of the room I saw the attending physician. I said, "I believe that your patient is dying." The attending looked surprised, saying, "He can't be dying, he doesn't have a terminal illness." As I regained my wits I stammered, "He has several: the myeloma, the progressive pneumonia, for starters." He responded, "The myeloma is responding to treatment and I don't have a clear diagnosis for the pneumonia, he can't be dying."

The patient apparently was undeterred by his lack of a diagnosis. He died two days later. The larger problem, Dr. Weissman writes, is all too common: "the failure of physicians to recognize when they are no longer in control of the dying process. The attending still felt he was in control of the cancer, in control of the pneumonia, in control of death, and perhaps in control of me. In fact he was not in control, and he could not or would not appreciate this fact to allow for a more timely recognition and approach to care to this dying patient."

Weissman writes that the answer is to teach physicians about the importance of hospice and palliative care and thereby educate them in the value of recognizing their own limitations.

Well and good. But patients may unwittingly contribute to the problem because they don't know what they want—or even what their options are. That is the conclusion of a thousand-patient study in Oregon. The research came after a ten-year debate in that state over whether to legalize physician-assisted suicide. There were legislative and court battles, as well as two highly controversial statewide referendum votes. If the public were to be aware of end-of-life care options anywhere, it would be in Oregon.

The survey gave patients a series of vignettes about a man named John who has cancer. John refuses chemotherapy. John loses the energy to eat and drink. John's breathing deteriorates until he needs a ventilator.

John writes his physician a note that reads, "Turn off the machine." The doctor obeys, but John lives on anyway. He asks his doctor to help him die right away. The doctor refuses but provides pain medication in doses large enough that, in addition to controlling John's pain, they might contribute to greater difficulty in breathing. Finally John dies peacefully.

At various steps in the survey's story, patients had to answer questions about what John could legally ask for and what the doctor could lawfully provide. Despite all the arguments in Oregon, years of headlines and strife over assisted suicide, the survey found people profoundly unaware of the law and their options.

On every question, hundreds of patients answered "don't know." Fewer than half of the survey respondents knew that mentally competent patients can tell their doctor to withdraw life-sustaining treatment such as ventilators. Only 41 percent answered correctly that it is legal for a doctor to give heavy pain medication even if it has the side effect of compromising breathing. Most stunning of all, 64 percent of the survey respondents said that euthanasia—in which a doctor gives a patient drugs that immediately end life—is legal. It is not legal; it is manslaughter.

What does this say about people who go to the effort to establish advance directives? They are more informed. They have made a greater effort to exert control over their care.

Yet their planning may be wasted energy, given that so many doctors do not bother to check to see whether patients have a directive in place. One study found that 70 percent of physicians failed even to determine whether dying patients wanted to be resuscitated in an emergency.

Worst of all, a physician who ignores an advance directive faces no consequences for that offense. State medical boards do not discipline doctors for this misconduct. And families, who might complain when their loved one's instructions are ignored, are too overwhelmed to do so.

That is what happened with Katherine Kemp Cross. No one explicitly chose not to hold doctors accountable for ignoring her directives, Dana said. She and her siblings simply had too much else on their minds.

"You're just stunned that you've lost your loved one. You're just not emotionally equipped to deal with what happened in the medical world. . . . You're in this cluster of grief with your siblings. And there is so much to do. You're sort of intimidated, too. And the person is gone, after all. It is such a shame."

No wonder so few people bother with advance directives. There's too little chance that they will make a difference.

* * *

ONE FOOTNOTE IS CRUCIAL about these legal instruments. They are not useful only to limit care. They can also make demands for aggressive treatment, which is equally valuable for patients who want that approach.

Thus far, discussion of advance directives has focused on how they are used to limit treatment at the end of life. That inclination reflects common public views. The Institute of Medicine cites a Gallup poll that found 90 percent of people, if they had less than six months to live, would want limited care at home rather than advanced medical intervention.

But that finding is no argument for ignoring the desires of the remaining 10 percent. Nor does it acknowledge those patients among the 90 percent who may change their minds when death draws near.

What is really important about advance directives—why more people ought to have them and why they ought to carry greater weight among doctors and hospitals—is that they transfer control of the dying process from the health-care providers to patients and their families.

In plainer terms, there is no one way to die, no correct method that will work for everyone. Rather, each person's life will close in a unique manner—and aligning that process with each person's values and wishes is a greater challenge because advance directives have so little effect. The goal is not to strengthen these documents because they limit care and bring on death. The point is to put the sick person in charge. Advance directives are not about dying faster, they are about living better—with control.

"EVERYTHING IN CONSUMER law for the past twenty-five years has been about empowerment," says Drew Edmondson, attorney general of Oklahoma and, until his term recently expired, president of the National Association of Attorneys General—the top law-enforcement officers of the fifty states. In a series of meetings involving the entire association membership, hospice experts and others led workshops exploring end-of-life-care issues. During the closed-door sessions, many in the gathering wept.

"Now we are approaching this as a consumer issue," explains Edmondson. "Will my pain be managed? Will my wishes be known and honored? Will I receive competent care?"

The answers, Edmondson suggests, are not what they need to be.

"Pain management? There's the lack of attention this subject is given in medical school and nursing schools. Doctors are trained to save life; they are not equipped to deal with death itself, and they are not focused on making death easy. Advance directives? They ought to carry the weight of statute. Instead, we have people not even checking to see if there is an advance directive in place. Also there is a certain fear of litigation that causes providers to err on the side of extraordinary care. Competency? Nearly fifty percent of all nursing-home residents today are in pain. To me, that's not competent care."

Edmondson's goal is to engage the fifty attorneys general on the issues so that they enlighten their states' medical regulators and legislators. "Between eighty and ninety percent of people express in polls that they would prefer to die at home, free from pain, attended by family and friends. You can flip that number and get what happens in the real world, with eighty percent in a health facility, in pain, absent friends and family."

The rights of the dying, Edmondson says, "are the number one consumer issue in the United States."

CHAPTER TWENTY-FOUR

DREAMS COMING TRUE

L iving well while dying gradually can be a noble task, especially if the days are made up of many small gifts. When a woman who has always loved choral music at long last receives voice lessons—taking them in the bed from which she will never rise—she and her teacher are not just cheating death, they are affirming life.

It happens with greater frequency now that dying has become a slow process. People have time to shape their days in ways that are meaningful to them. The wishes they have, the desires and compulsions, are unique to each person. Ironically, the process somewhat resembles a wedding: The bride-to-be selects details about the ceremony, clothes, invitations, and more, all intended to express some resonant family symbolism, special friendship, or heartfelt hope for the marriage ahead. And it is never the same for any two brides. Last wishes have a similar quality, expressing not an illness or a decline but a personality and a life.

THOMAS ROLLERSON LEARNED these lessons the hard way, but then put his experience to constructive use for others' sake.

In 1994 Thomas's longtime partner, Timothy Scott Palmer, was fighting renal failure due to AIDS. At the time, many of the medicines that now curtail that disease were not widely available. Timm, thirty-four, was a great optimist, a laughing man with a ready smile, and an aspiring filmmaker. One of his favorite performers was Robin Williams.

When Timm's illness was well advanced, he and Thomas went to see

Williams star in the film *Mrs. Doubtfire*. Timm was severely dehydrated, requiring him to drink water constantly, and his weakened immune system required distilled water. But the theater would not let him in with his own water bottle. In terms of society's treatment of people with AIDS, it was a less enlightened time.

"It was humiliating," Thomas said. "He was there literally in his pajamas. But he was denied access. For me, I was broken. I couldn't do anything for him."

Then Thomas had the brainstorm of contacting 20th Century-Fox to see if he could obtain an advance videotape of the movie. They said yes, expedited its copying, and released it for Timm.

"He was blown away that they would do that for him," Thomas said. "That was huge. The industry that he had aspired to acknowledged him. To see him impressed, and laughing again, this was medicine like no other."

Thomas spoke with one of Timm's nurses about what had happened, which led to another idea: "What can I do for the other patients? What other dreams are there?"

Soon he was busy learning other patients' wishes and doing what he could to fulfill them. By the time Timm died on April 19, 1994, Thomas had found a new life purpose. "I wanted to do something with the love, and not the anger or the grief. I have a choice. And I chose the love."

Thomas formed the Dream Foundation, a Santa Barbara–based non-profit company that helps dying people realize their dearest remaining desires. The organization has fulfilled about six thousand dreams so far. Most are surprisingly modest.

"Yesterday I spent time with a woman with fourteen grandchildren. She has a twin bed. She wants a queen bed so the grandchildren can get in with her."

Another bedridden patient did not have the use of his arms. But he was eager to read, to occupy his still active brain. "We found an electronic piece of equipment to help him, a page-turner machine."

Some people want hearing aids, "so they can hear their loved ones' voices more clearly before they die." Others want trips to places like Disney World—not for themselves, but for their children. "If these people are low-income, they have already been profoundly impacted financially by the illness," Thomas said. "They may have never been on vacation before."

One young man with cancer and a powerful love for his girlfriend knew that chemotherapy would make him sterile. The foundation fronted eight hundred dollars so he could bank his sperm. Another man went with his son to the Napa Valley wine country. Still another wanted to attend his son's graduation, despite his severely limited mobility.

"The best ones are when dreams are resolution-based," Thomas said. "That's the ultimate gift we can give anyone, a sense of peace." Those dreams often involve bringing family members together, flying them in from around the country to resolve old issues and say last good-byes. "Often we hear from the dreamers, 'All right, it's okay now.'"

The longer he works in the foundation, Thomas said, the more he believes the actual dreams are secondary to less tangible things the dreamers receive. "They come to us with hope. After all, our dreams are what propel us out of bed in the morning. At that stage in their illness, they have been so filled with fear and disappointment. The first thing we give them is listening. Sometimes they die before we get the dream arranged, even though we move swiftly. But it's all right, because we make it okay to dream. It's difficult for people to ask for anything. They've been humbled by the care they've received. We are validating that it's okay to ask. Just knowing that the dream might happen gives us hope."

Having a dream to live for sometimes brings a resurgence of health, too, Thomas said. "Right now we're working with a woman, an artist her whole life, who never got to do an art show. We are working on doing that art show for her. She has completely rebounded, because she has a purpose."

Other organizations also help dying people realize their dreams—most notably, the Make-A-Wish Foundation, which has granted 127,000 wishes since its founding in 1980. That organization serves children exclusively, while the Dream Foundation considers dreamers of all ages. In both cases the idea is to address people's needs that are distinctly nonmedical.

Also in both cases, there is a dangerous temptation to believe that philanthropic groups can somehow fill the gap between what dying people need today and what they actually receive. These organizations cannot do that job, not only because they don't have the money but also because most people do not want miracles. They want competence. People do not want special treatment. They want control.

"Every being," Thomas said, "every single being deserves to die in comfort and dignity, and in as much peace as possible."

The Dream Foundation shows how a little compassion and generosity can make all sorts of final chapters possible. As important as the foundation's work is, all it takes for people to have their wishes answered is decent medical care, strong self-determination, and some loving help.

Here are stories of some people who prove the point—not by how they died but by how they lived.

WILLIAM HANLEY was a dapper man with a devil-may-care attitude toward life. His children said he was a reincarnation of Jay Gatsby, only without all the money. Still, whatever car William owned at any given time he would always customize by adding the largest air horns he could find—long pipes built for the biggest of tractor-trailers. All around Ligonier, Pennsylvania, people recognized the blaring blast of his car horns. William's other love was shooting; he had been a skeet champion in his younger days. He displayed his handsome guns in glass cases placed prominently in his home. The cases held trophies and ribbons he'd won over the years. Even more than shooting, William enjoyed a good party.

In 1997 William was diagnosed with prostate cancer. Surgery and radiation brought only a temporary reprieve. The cancer spread to his bones. One day in early 1999 his doctor told him there was nothing more they could do. William was dying. He responded by going home, mixing up a frosty jug of gin and tonics, grabbing his daughter and her husband, and driving out to his gravesite. There, standing before a stone bearing his birth year of 1924 and a blank place for the year of his death, they had cocktails. He even posed for a photo with one hand on the stone. In the picture he is smiling, giving a thumbs-up.

The following Memorial Day weekend, hospice workers called William's family to say that the end was near. His children flew in from around the country and gathered at his bedside. On the third day he awakened from a morphine haze to say that he knew why they had come but he was not ready to die just yet. He had something to do first.

Four weeks later, in a skeet competition in Virginia, William shot twenty-five straight clays—a perfect score. That feat, which few people can do when healthy, won him the senior division championship. He went on that summer to win several other competitions, traveling as far west as Arizona.

By winter William's health had turned again, though he continued to entertain people from his bed right to the end. In 2000 William died at home in the care of the local hospice. At the end of his memorial service, there were no mournful tolling bells. Instead, just after the final prayer, William's son drove his father's car to the church door and let loose a blast from those infernal horns. The entire congregation laughed.

．　　　．　　　．

AT THE OTHER END of the socioeconomic spectrum lives Carole Gaudreault. Her home is a railroad-style apartment on U.S. 4 in Enfield, New Hampshire. It is a somewhat hardscrabble place. Carole never finished high school, so the best job she ever had was at a nearby ball bearing plant. Now seventy-two, she receives $431 from Social Security, $153 from a pension, $110 in food stamps, and $7 from New Hampshire's welfare program, a total of $701 per month.

Carole's windows are filled with plants. Ceramic cats cover her dresser and tables. The TV is nearly always on, turned up loud. Finches and a pair of lovebirds named Hekyll and Jekyll maintain a running commentary on the room's activity. Frisky, Rebel, and other house cats periodically prowl by to see if anyone has inadvertently left a birdcage open.

Carole spends her days in a hospital bed, with a bar overhead to help pull herself upright. She is making an afghan for one of her fifteen grandchildren or seven great-grandchildren. The pattern is complicated, but she can knit, purl, and crochet without interrupting the conversation.

"August twenty-ninth, 1994, that was the day they took off my right breast," she recalls. "Thirteen lymph nodes they counted, and eight was cancerous."

After chemotherapy, Carole enjoyed several years of good health. Now she has tumors on her spine. Yet her mood is consistently upbeat.

"That chemo? I didn't lose my hair or nothing. When I went for my MRI, people were saying how can you stand two hours in that thing? Didn't bother me a bit. You can listen to the music while they're doing it. They asked me what I want. I told them: country and western."

Carole says her condition is helped by optimism. "My left leg is giving me a lot of trouble, but I get around all right." She searches for the remote among the blankets, then quiets the television. "I think a lot of it is that I don't let it bother me."

Carole also receives comprehensive home health care. Fourteen different prescriptions clutter the bedside table. A pillbox organizes her medications into morning, noon, evening, and bedtime dosages. A purse-size computerized device calibrates the drip of pain medicine into a tube permanently fixed to her hip.

"We've named that Robert," she jokes, picking up the machine and demonstrating its functions. "The hospice nurse runs this, but I about could do it myself by now. See? I've had 110.6 milliliters so far today."

If the machine failed, Carole knows it would mean agony. "I would be suffering, you bet. But I haven't had no problems. Or if I have pain I can't stand, I just press 'dose' and in about four minutes I can feel everything getting dull."

Being home is essential to maintaining a positive attitude, Carole says. It keeps her connected with her family, her pets, and her sense of autonomy. "No way I would go to a home now. I'd kill myself first. I've had friends go in a home. They say your life is not your own."

Carole has glowing things to say about her caretakers. "That hospice nurse, she is one good, nice lady. And all the girls that come in and wash me up, they're real good, too."

But she reserves her highest praise for the man who quiets her pain, Dennis Coombs, M.D. Sometimes her gratitude veers toward being a crush.

"He is a good doctor, I know that. He's very grandfathery, though I think I am older than he is. I joked with him, 'Too bad you're married.'"

"I'm old-fashioned, hands-on," Dr. Coombs says. "When Carole comes in to the office, I'll give her a hug. She's a great lady. In fact, Carole is one of my favorite patients because her attitude under the worst crisis is so positive."

She is also seriously ill, he says. "People in this condition experience progressive uncontrolled nerve pain as they basically become paralyzed. The tumor invades the nerve roots, spreads into the canal, and grows. The pain escalates out of control."

He could sever part of her spinal cord to stop the pain, but it would mean paralysis. He could use a full-body drug like morphine, but the dosage would quell her alertness and function. Robert, the device on her hip, is a sustained local anesthetic, numbing a fixed area much like the epidural pain relief some women receive during labor. Under this protocol patients live longer and function better; when the disease prevails, their suffering is brief. "They'll get a metastasis to the brain, suffer a seizure, and they're gone."

Until then, patients' high quality of life is equally rewarding for the physician, he adds. "A lot of people think of it as some sort of service. It's not a service. It is a privilege and a gift when you help people."

Coombs had a distinguished career—research, clinical work, department chairmanships at major medical schools. After losing a fortune investing in a medical-instrument company, he returned to patient care.

"It has been sort of a gift to be doing this," he says. There are problems with health insurers, patients who distrust doctors, policies in government, and health-care institutions that consider pain control a low priority. "You put in a lot of effort and time to get it right. These patients become like close friends."

Meanwhile, Carole celebrates her granddaughter's marriage. She visits with her sister, plays with her pets. All of it would be impossible without effective attention to her pain.

Of course, Carole's story cannot have a happy ending. Her medical care is being provided through hospice, which means she and Dr. Coombs have acknowledged that she has less than six months to live.

"I know I'm not going to get better, but I'm not suffering. From the waist down, pretty soon I am going to be paralyzed. They thought it would happen by December or January. Well, here it is March. The doctors think it's because I get up and move around and never wallow in self-pity."

Carole has a wheelchair for the days ahead, but until then she has put tennis balls on the legs of her walker so she can move faster. "Look, I've got this. I can't stop it. I'm going to have to learn to live with it.

"I can't complain. . . . Anything I need, the nicest people, the care I've had. And my granddaughter is just a shout away. This room, though"—she waves a hand at the clutter of papers, the overgrown plants, the seeds her birds have spilled from their cages onto the rug, and she laughs—"this I have *got* to clean."

As a visitor leaves her room, Carole turns the television volume back up. It's midday, the soaps are on. Her favorite program? *One Life to Live*.

CAROLE'S EXPERIENCE embodies how good care, respect, and sustained independence can provide a fulfilling last chapter of life. The story of Andy Waller, a trucker from Oklahoma City, builds on this idea by showing that such care can never come too late.

In 1980 Andy was finishing an unloading job when a car fell on him. He was thirty-two. During his immediate care, he received forty units of blood, a huge volume; he survived but was paralyzed from the waist down. Later complications landed him in the hospital, where a nurse was struck by Andy's positive attitude. They stayed in touch, they shared a home, they married.

"I was really impressed with his personality and strength of character," said Stephanie Waller. "He was in a wheelchair, but he was not sedentary in the least little bit."

She kept handy a photo of Andy refinishing the kitchen cabinets. He's angling in his chair for better leverage with the electric sander. He learned to drive using hand controls. Adding to children from a previous relationship, and despite his paralysis, Andy fathered two more. Years went by and Andy was a loving husband to Stephanie. Often they buzzed each other's pager with the return number of 222-2222, their way of saying, "I'm thinking of you."

On Thanksgiving Day 2001, Andy was smoking a turkey when he found a kidney stone in his urine pouch. Within hours he became sick. Doctors found that Andy had hepatitis C, likely a result of his massive transfusion twenty-one years earlier. His liver failed swiftly, and Andy rapidly became sicker.

He did not want to die, Stephanie said. "He fought. He wouldn't sign any advance directives. Not till the very end, and then only to say that I would decide when to let him go."

Andy's medical team fought, too, employing hydration tools and increasingly sophisticated drugs. For Stephanie, the career nurse, these efforts were futile and everyone knew it. "You're watching doctors trying to keep people alive," she said with dismay. "It's not what we're doing *for* the patient but what we're doing *to* the patient. They're afraid to say there's nothing we can do, especially because the family clings to any hope."

Andy turned the corner first. He reminded Stephanie, "There are no wheelchairs in heaven."

In early February they decided to bring Andy home. Insurance did not cover the ambulance "because it wasn't an emergency," Stephanie said. They used an ambulance anyway, but as far as the insurer was concerned, "I guess we could have thrown him in the back of a pickup or something."

On February 22 Stephanie was out doing an errand when her pager buzzed. The return number was 222-2222.

"That was the last time," she remembered. "Pretty soon after that he was comatose." The nurse in her checked to be certain. "If you lifted up his eyelids, the eyes were rolled back."

Loved ones began to gather. His older children, his kids with Stephanie. They crowded into the room. His brother-in-law, his niece, Stephanie's mother. More and more people stood by Andy's side. Half a dozen friends, other relatives. Remembering that day, Stephanie needed a moment to give a total count—eighteen, plus the big family mutt, Tom-Girl. They held one another, they told stories, they laughed long and loud.

In the middle of it all Stephanie glanced over at her comatose husband. "Andy was smiling. Grinning."

The next day Andy's breathing slowed, and Stephanie climbed into bed beside him. "The whole time I had my arms around him. I whispered in his ear, 'I will love you forever. Take that with you.'

"There was none of the usual gasping at the end. He just eased down, slowed. It was the weirdest thing. I have attended a lot of deaths. I have never seen an easier one."

SMILING IN A COMA is one sure sign of a peaceful exit. But Margaret Alexander gave even more uplifting evidence: laughing and dancing.

Margaret lived nearly all her life in Longmeadow, Massachusetts. Only five feet three inches tall, she was nonetheless considered a noticeably attractive woman. She married a man who told friends he had fallen in love with her voice. Bernard Strempel proposed on their third date; she became pregnant on their honeymoon.

Margaret loved romantic, jazzy music—Frank Sinatra, Nat King Cole, Herb Alpert. She also loved to laugh and could make jokes in even the darkest situations. She and Bernard had four children.

When she turned seventy, Margaret started having stomach problems. She ignored them until a neighbor who is a nurse persuaded her to get examined. A tumor had encroached throughout her abdomen. Immediately she underwent major medical interventions, from surgery to insertion of a hockey-puck-size chemotherapy device directly in her gut.

Her oncologist "didn't have a whole lot of personality," recalls Margaret's daughter Sandy, so she was always trying to get him to joke around. He brought in some interns one day, asking if she minded. "She said, 'Help yourself, everyone else does,'" Sandy recalls. Margaret was on a strict diet, but she hid a granola bar in her eyeglasses case and snuck it when no one was looking.

The disease continued its march, but at least the interventions bought her family some time. "If she had died within that first month, it would have been so much harder," Sandy says. "There's little you can do when someone's dying of cancer. Putting a cloth on her face, getting ice chips. It sounds small, but it's such a privilege to do that. It's a wonderful opportunity to give your love. I think she was touched, too, by how we cared for her. Like, 'Wow, they're doing all this for me.' But really it was a gift to yourself, and it would make it easier to handle after because you have no regrets."

Nobody wanted to talk about Margaret's decline, evident as it was in her thinning face and swollen belly. Finally in June Bernard asked the doctor, who said she had about a week to live.

The family gathered at home, Margaret in her bedroom unconscious before a Red Sox game on the TV. "I went in there," Sandy says, "and you think she's out of it. And she announces, 'That pitcher Derek Lowe sucks, they've got to get rid of him.'"

One morning Margaret had a pronouncement. "Tomorrow is the big day," she said. So she wanted to have a party, right away.

"She got out of bed, put on a sundress," Sandy recalls. "She was very, very weak—you have to picture it—but she's putting on lipstick. She knew she was going and she wanted to go out on a happy note. Then she said she wanted a martini. My sister-in-law was concerned that it would be bad for her. I was like, God, she's dying, why not?"

Margaret began telling jokes nonstop. She insisted they put on her favorite music. Then Margaret and a nephew went out on the back deck. While Tony Bennett sang, they danced.

"It was a beautiful moment," Sandy remembers. "She totally seemed pain-free."

Later, back in bed, Margaret sat visiting with a favorite niece. "I was cooking, and I could hear them laughing all day," Sandy says. When she entered her mother's room, Margaret murmured, "Tomorrow is the big day. I understand everything now. There'll be three lights, and it'll be time for me to go."

Sandy slept beside her that night. Margaret kept waking, asking what time it was. She also began talking about dead family members who she would be seeing. "I just held her and hugged her," Sandy says. "She went limp, and said, 'Okay.' Right after that she went into the coma."

The family gathered at Margaret's bedside, holding her hands. She took three deep breaths. "When she took that last one, her face was really peaceful." And she was gone.

The prevailing sentiment that morning was not sadness, Sandy says. "It was almost like a sense of elation. We were smiling. Partly it was relief that it's over, partly that she would've wanted us to be that way."

On the way to the funeral days later, the family retold Margaret's spiciest jokes. "In the limo we were in hysterics, laughing," Sandy recalls. "The driver probably thought we were crazy. Then we arrived, and it was, 'We've got to clean up our act. Everyone out there is so glum.' But you see, they hadn't lived it."

Afterward there was a party at a relative's house. "We got cases of beer," Sandy says. "And we played all kinds of jazz tunes. The kind my mom loved."

IF THESE STORIES OFFER EVIDENCE of how last wishes and pleasures can persist right up to the final moment of life, then Lorraine Hoover shows how they can continue beyond that point.

Born in New York City in 1920, Lorraine always had a rebellious streak. She met Richard Barstow, a doctor from Norfolk, Connecticut, fifteen years her senior, and married him forty days later.

Lorraine often raised eyebrows in their small town. Protestants and Catholics in that era practiced a self-imposed segregation, yet she befriended a Catholic named Patricia Quinlan. One Christmas Eve during the Vietnam War she staged a peace vigil on the steps of the Congregational church, upsetting parishioners. Lorraine embraced feminism and the environmental movement. She made arrangements for an Ethiopian exchange student to live with them in Norfolk. When his family was slaughtered while he was studying in America, she became his surrogate mother.

A melanoma in her neck prompted surgery in 1985, but Lorraine had clear health afterward. Then in 1997 the melanoma returned. "They always say if it comes back, you're a dead duck," says her son John.

The diagnosis came in late October. Lorraine's decline began at once. She called her five children together for Thanksgiving but was mentally absent much of the time. "She looked like a ghost," John says. "We were all walking around sobbing but trying to be all sunny around her."

By then Richard was in a nursing home with dementia. He kept forgetting who was dying, his wife or his long-dead mother. "In the world of senility, it made perfect sense," John says. "It was very poignant, the last time she visited him."

After Thanksgiving Lorraine inexplicably regained awareness of her surroundings. She arranged for hospice care. Her daughter Noel took advantage of the Family and Medical Leave Act, moving in as a caretaker.

One day Lorraine assigned John and his wife, Kate, a task. "I have never wanted to support the mortuary mafia," she told them. "They make people spend at their most vulnerable times. I don't want anything to do with them."

Kate did the homework. They were allowed to care for the body and move it, provided they had proper permits. Lorraine approved. In the following weeks she shrank, though, her body covered with bumps, while her children gathered close.

Yet John remembers the time fondly. "You get this incredible privilege to accompany a loved one on their journey. There's a lot of hard work—my sister did most of it. But we didn't any of us have unresolved issues. Everybody was able to visit and have wonderful talks with her."

On January 1, 1998, Lorraine's children knelt by her bed, while outside a storm tossed the night. Someone suggested giving Lorraine some space for a few minutes, and they left the room. Moments later her breathing stopped.

"There was a certain amount of rejoicing that was totally appropriate," John recalls. "Then, of course, she's dead. It was bittersweet, tears of joy and tears of sorrow."

A hospice volunteer helped Lorraine's daughters wash and dress her. "And there she lay on her bed that night and the next day," John says. "Resting. The window open a bit, the thermostat in the room turned off." Family members entered the room often. "Some people believe that it takes some time after the last breath for the spirit to leave the body. Mother's spirit had time to linger. To take its leave. Her death had time to sink into us. This is missing from conventional modern death. For us it felt natural."

Lorraine's sons and sons-in-law built her a box of rough-cut wood. Fortunately, one son-in-law is a skilled carpenter, because John said he and his brother "were making a fairly major botch of that box." The finished coffin had a strong scent of fresh fir.

Someone thought to line the box with Lorraine's down comforter. A grandchild added a teddy bear. "Many other tokens—notes, keepsakes, drawings, photographs, carvings—were tenderly placed in the box over the next several days," John says. "There are all of these decisions you can make if you're doing this yourself, so much symbolism, and you can express care."

The grandchildren were not put off by mortuary tasks, John says. "They were exposed to it all, but not pressured. There was a show on the Discovery Channel about fighter jets, which was perfect for the boys. But when it came time we said, 'Guys, we're going to move Nana now.' They all came to the door to watch. They were curious."

The experience of lifting his mother's body is "too personal and intimate to put into words," John says, but it was "another in a whole series of acts in the process of caring for one's own dead that—once taken—hold love, meaning, sorrow, healing."

The next few days were more typical, John recalls: flowers, food, family arriving. But there were two huge differences that may have been connected. First, sibling conflicts were somehow put entirely aside. Second, "there was a superb focus and comfort: Mother was in the garage."

Candles remained lit all around her box. A handmade wreath lay on top, with seeds to attract birds. The family chose not to remove the garage contents, though, the woodpile and garden implements. "Mom was surrounded by the modest tools and possessions of life and activity, not somber brocade draperies and plush carpeting. This is precisely what she would have wanted."

People kept visiting the garage. With "so many chances to say good-bye," John recalls, "the bitter kept fading and the sweet became more intense."

The family held a service outdoors. One aunt with more traditional views gave a Bible reading. "It was a perfect ingredient," John says. They drove the box to a crematory. They wrote the only check of the entire process, for eighty dollars. They said good-bye and drove home.

But soon Lorraine's children realized their work was incomplete. Richard kept asking for his wife and needed to be reminded that she had died. So they arranged a formal service.

"It was great," John recalls. "This was the church where he baptized all of his children, where he was married. We got my father down, and it turned out to be so important. Patricia Quinlan was there. There were poems, a eulogy. The Ethiopian exchange student, he came back, too. He's now a professor in Southern California, and he wanted to speak about her."

A counterculture wake and two memorials made perfect sense for his mother, John maintains. "Both forms of closure are important. It was great."

LORRAINE BARSTOW MANAGED to exert her preferences and personality beyond the end of her life. For younger people who are dying slowly, even greater deeds are possible.

Alan Jakubek was a photographer from Washington State. He was handsome in an outdoorsy way. Though he always had a sweetheart on his arm, Alan was commitment-shy. He said he needed freedom to follow his artistic impulses. That way of life worked for thirty-five years, until he met Caroline Crawford, a woman from Staten Island, New York, who was eleven years younger. He fell hard.

A woman approached Caroline at a party. "So, you're the one who tamed the wolf," she said. Alan and Caroline married in 1996, and in 2000 Caroline delivered a baby boy, Carl. Alan was rapturous and immediately wanted another child.

Yet Alan's mood changed in the months after Carl's birth. He developed an uncharacteristically short temper. He lost interest in work—something previously unheard-of—and even skipped a few photo assignments. In early 2001 Alan went to a doctor, who diagnosed depression over the life changes caused by Carl's arrival. He prescribed Zoloft.

Caroline didn't believe it. She insisted that Alan go back to the doctor. While he was in the examining room, Alan had a seizure. He was rushed to a hospital, where tests and an emergency biopsy revealed he had more than a dozen lymphoma lesions in his brain. It was a rare cancer, and a bad one.

But Alan was only forty-three, and had a positive attitude. He would start chemotherapy in a few weeks. When a doctor warned that the process would make him sterile, Alan made five trips to a sperm bank. "We had always talked about having two children. But this poor man has a hole cut in his head from the biopsy, and he's trying to ejaculate every morning at nine A.M." Caroline went with him to the facility, and she laughs at the memory. "Let's just say he approached everything with a playful attitude."

But after he produced his final vial, Alan grew serious. "No matter what happens to me," Caroline recalls him saying, "I really want you to have another baby. I don't want you and Carl to be alone."

Caroline had her answer ready. "I promise you that I will."

Alan underwent two kinds of chemotherapy, then a stem-cell transplant that brought an apparent remission. It lasted only two months. He and Caroline found leading specialists in his cancer in Oregon and went to them for care. He endured radiation. The disease marched on. Finally the Oregon doctors said Alan would live only a few more months.

At Caroline's next ovulation, she was inseminated. Alan came to the appointment. She called the syringe "the turkey baster," and when the procedure was over Alan joked, "Honey, I hope I'm better than that."

Six days later Caroline was at work when she took a pregnancy test that gave a faint positive. "I was weak, I was so excited," she says. "I called him at home and whispered it to him." Later they agreed it was far too early to tell anyone, "but when I went upstairs I heard him dialing the phone." Alan called his sister, a friend, another relative—in all, eight people he entrusted with his delight. Alan accompanied Caroline to her first obstetric appointment, which included an ultrasound. "When he saw the fetal blob, and the little tiny heart beating, he was excited, yes, pretty excited."

The joy was short-lived. On July 24 Alan relapsed. On August 13 the oncologist said they could manage his pain, but there was nothing else to be done. What does that mean? Alan asked. Six months? Nine?

"A couple of weeks," Caroline recalls. "They said a couple of weeks. I was seven weeks pregnant."

That night they went out to dinner, had steak sandwiches; Alan drank a few beers. They planned a last trip. A few days later they stayed in the best suite at a mountainside inn. They ordered room service, and Alan had five desserts. They took a bath together.

"It was heart-wrenching for me," Caroline recalls. "He was losing weight, he was starting to lose the use of his hand and right leg. I could see he was getting one hundred percent worse every day."

Alan led Caroline out onto the balcony to enjoy the view. "Let's pick out a name," she said. "Shhh, honey," he replied, "we've got lots of time for that."

"There was a long pause," Caroline recalls, "then he said, 'Maybe we don't. No, maybe we don't.'"

If it was a girl, they agreed on a family name, Elizabeth, with the middle name Grace "for all the grace and mercy shown to us," Caroline says. A boy would be Peter, after Alan's close friend of that name, with the middle name of Gustav, after Caroline's grandfather.

By the time of Caroline's twelve-week appointment, Alan was living in an inpatient hospice facility. He told everyone there that he and his wife were expecting. "I don't know what we were thinking," she recalls, "and I certainly didn't want to do it alone. But I was hoping the pregnancy would keep him focused and hopeful, and believing this would all work out."

Alan died on September 5, 2002. Caroline was three months pregnant. "Carrying a baby got me through those first six months," she recalls.

Elizabeth Grace was born on March 25, 2003.

"She's got Alan's big blue eyes, and his smile. I see him every time I look at her. It's him looking out at me."

Elizabeth has been an easy baby, Caroline says. She was baptized on what would have been her parents' seventh wedding anniversary. "I wanted to do something to make it less horrible. Alan's family came, which was great of them. We were sad but also celebrating her."

Elizabeth plays happily with her big brother and loves to look at photographs of her father. "A lot of people said Alan and I were crazy. But now it is so wonderful that we have this new part of Alan alive. She is the most amazing kid I have ever seen. She's a complete gift to this whole family. And to everyone around us, too.

"So how is that for a last wish being granted? It was the most life-affirming thing I could give him. Turns out I gave it to a lot of people."

CHAPTER TWENTY-FIVE

THE FINAL CARESS

The last sensation a dying person feels ought to be loving: a caress, an embrace, a nurturing that makes the passage out of life as gentle and unfrightening as possible. For people whose heart stops in a hospital, the reality could not be further from that ideal.

First the person discovering the patient's condition immediately presses an emergency-call button on the wall. This is known as "calling a code," and it summons on the run as many as eight people—cardiac and emergency doctors, nurses, an anesthesiologist. That first person begins a series of fierce compressions on the patient's chest: one hand atop the other, placed against the breastbone and jammed downward. The intent is to push blood out of the heart so the brain continues to receive oxygen. Every few pumps, the caregiver provides two breaths to the patient.

The code team arrives. Over the patient's face the anesthesiologist hooks a mask connected to a bellows so respiration help continues. To restart the heart, the patient receives between fifty and one hundred joules of electric current, what a conscious person would feel as a harsh jolt. Just before the switch is thrown, the head of the code team calls, "Clear," so the crew can pull away and avoid a nasty shock. A shot of adrenaline comes next.

Meanwhile, another team member works to collect a blood sample to find out how acidic the patient's blood has become—the more acidic, the worse off the patient is. With circulation stopped, however, getting a sample is difficult; arteries lie flaccid like the paper wrapper of a drinking straw. The quick solution—and in a code everything must be quick—is to go after the big artery in the patient's groin. So his legs are splayed wide, and the team member jabs in a syringe. It's rare to strike oil on the first try. To improve the odds of repeat attempts, the doctor leaves the first syringe in place to indicate where not to jab. Often a patient will have three or four syringes sticking out of his groin before a blood sample is rushed off to the lab.

Remember, all this time the patient's heart has been stopped. If his brain does not receive oxygen within six minutes, it begins to die. Brain tissue does not regenerate, so losses are beyond recovery. If the heart restarts, the patient will move on to the ICU and life on a ventilator. In time, doctors will sort out the degree of damage to the brain and other vital organs.

Codes routinely run longer than six minutes, though. If the patient is particularly young or strong, the team might try an even further intervention—cracking the chest. A physician slices open the patient's skin, reaches in, and manually massages the heart to force circulation. There is no anesthesia.

Such assaultive medicine is permitted in large measure because of unrealistic public expectations. One doctor performed an odd but significant study in this regard. She and a team of researchers reviewed every episode of one season of the TV shows *ER* and *Chicago Hope*, as well as fifty episodes of *Rescue 911*, tracking their use of CPR. Seventy-five percent of the TV characters who received this treatment survived, 67 percent recovered to leave the hospital, and all of the survivors recovered fully.

That's TV; reality is not so pleasant. Study results vary, but people in cardiac arrest outside of hospitals have survival rates as low as 2 percent. In hospitals, the rate can run as low as 1 percent. Of those, the recovery data is even more discouraging. As many as half of these patients' brains have spent too long without oxygen. That is one of the ways that society winds up with thirty-five thousand people living in a persistent vegetative state. *Living* might also be a generous word for the unmoving, unconscious, machine-sustained existence they and their families endure.

It is not unreasonable to believe that a person with a stopped heart is already dead. Yet running a code is the defined standard of care for in-hospital cardiac arrests, and has been since a Massachusetts Supreme Court decision in 1998. Many doctors believe codes to be painful and futile. But they and their hospitals may be held liable for negligence if they fail to perform every possible procedure on a patient with a stopped heart. It is hard to imagine a deathbed experience further from a caress.

There is a means of preventing a code. It is called a DNR order, for "Do not resuscitate." Some people misunderstand a DNR as a decree to stop efforts to keep them alive. That is not the case. All a DNR establishes is that when the patient's heart finally stops, he or she does not receive CPR or ventilator care. A DNR means "do all you can to keep me alive, but when I am dead, then let me go."

For the person approaching death, it seems a sensible line to draw. Yet neither a patient nor a family member can issue a DNR. It is a medical order, entered on the patient's chart with a physician's signature of approval.

Obtaining a doctor's permission sounds easy. But taking that step could have unintended and undesirable side effects. One study of people with and without DNR orders, in New York City and Washington, D.C., asked their satisfaction with the care they received as death neared. The survey shows that patients' satisfaction did not change much based on the severity of their illness, nor on how painful their disease was. Instead, researchers found an unexpected cause of differences in patient satisfaction: DNRs.

"Patients who had DNR orders and were treated by the house-staff service gave their physicians especially low quality ratings compared with all other patients," the study reports.

The number of interviews was too small for researchers to determine exactly why this was so, but the data prompted several theories. Perhaps "physicians simply lose interest in dying patients, and patients with DNR orders are likely to be the victims of this lack of interest. Others apparently believe that patients with DNR orders are abandoned by the staff."

Whatever the reason, the outcome is the same: At a time in life when people ought to have the most autonomy, the maximum control over their medical treatment, they turn out to have almost none. And if they exert their will and obtain a physician's permission for the treatment plan they want, they may have to accept lower-quality care as a consequence.

DIRE AS THE SITUATION IS, discussion about advance directives can be misleading because it concerns only a subset of larger issues. Ignored legal instructions exemplify the extent to which people's medical wishes could be better fulfilled. But dying is only partly a biological event. It is also a social event, an economic one, and, above all for many people, a spiritual one. Indeed, the closer death comes, the less medicine is a factor at all. Eventually treatments become ineffective at changing the course of events, while other concerns come to the fore.

Of course a dying person wants excellent medical care up to and including the final second. But that is a mere fraction of one's overall needs. Unique as each person is, end-of-life-care scholars see many common elements to the wishes of people who are dying:

- They want to know what their disease is, how it works, at what pace and intensity they can expect it to overcome them.

- They want to know what to expect in their ability to function—what they will lose, how fast, and in what order.

- They want to know how much it will hurt, and what options they have for minimizing suffering.

- They want hope, even though its definition changes over time. What begins as hope for a cure may become hope for more time, then hope for continued function, then hope for having loved ones near, then hope for experiencing a quiet passage.

- People want to mourn their own death. They know better than anyone what they are losing, and want to grieve those losses.

- They want to protect their loved ones. They want to resolve relationships whenever possible. They want to minimize the grief they cause their families. They do not want to be a burden, nor bankrupt their spouse and family. They want reassurance that their loved ones will be all right when it is over.

- They want to know in advance about symptoms like shortness of breath so they can face problems before they become severe.

- They want to make informed decisions. They want to be realistic without being fatalistic. They want to believe that the medical team is doing a good job.

- They want their doctors and nurses to see them not as an object manifesting a disease but as a complete person who has a life entirely beyond the present illness.

- As their hair falls out, their weight declines, and their skin tone changes, they do not want to become ugly.

- They want last wishes honored, whether it is a meal or a trip or a conversation. They want to stay home.

- They do not want to be bored, grimly dripping away their last hours. They want company, when they have the energy, because for the dying there is no pain greater than loneliness.

- One thing they want that medical science is not equipped to provide is spiritual peace. Whatever their belief system, they want their life's final days to be enriched by that faith.

- They want to know that after their death their body will be treated with dignity, and in a way that reflects their values.

How well are these needs met?

Joanne Lynn, M.D., of Americans for Better Care of the Dying in Washington, D.C., provides a fair accounting: "In our system, it is easier to get open heart surgery than Meals on Wheels, easier to get antibiotics than eyeglasses, and certainly easier to get emergency medical care aimed at rescue than sustaining, supportive care."

An article in the *Annals of Internal Medicine* concurs: "This elevation of the science of medicine above the humanity of the patient is a serious problem that cannot be resolved without changes in the organization and culture of the hospital and the active support of hospital leaders.

"It is easier to keep patients alive on ventilators than it is to grapple with withdrawing support, and it is easier to define success in terms of life and death than to try to determine the quality of life that is meaningful to an individual patient," write the article's physician-authors.

All true—but again the focus is primarily clinical. One study, of nearly one thousand terminal patients who were interviewed twice in their final months, concludes that an emphasis on strictly medical requirements eclipsed patients' other important needs.

"Remarkably, no detailed comprehensive framework has emerged to guide and evaluate policy and care interventions" the study reports. "Instead, much of recent attention to end-of-life care focuses on selected physical aspects of suffering, such as pain, or on selected aspects of decision-making, such as the do-not-resuscitate order, which may be important to physicians but are of less concern to patients. Other important aspects of patients' experience have been marginalized."

People in this research project had the usual deficits in their care: half lived with moderate or severe pain, 71 percent were short of breath, many were incontinent and depressed.

But the study's concern was nonmedical issues. Patients were asked

212 · LAST RIGHTS

dozens of questions to determine how they felt—not physically but emotionally. Could they speak freely about the end of their lives? Had they settled their personal relationships? Did they have anyone to talk to? Were they angry, distressed, or bitter? Did they have someone who showed them love and affection? Did they have important projects they wanted to finish? Had their doctor or nurse given clear explanations of what was going on? Were these clinicians respectful? Had they had sufficient access to any specialists they might have needed to see? Had their illness been a financial hardship? Did they have a faith or a religious community that supported them? Were they in much pain?

The mere existence of a study that asks such questions is a sign of progress. The well-being of people who are dying is more than a medical issue; curiosity about nonbiological aspects is a step in the right direction.

The patients' answers were interesting, too. First, the level of their pain and distress was not subjective after all; it was measurable. Second, the high importance patients gave to nonmedical issues highlights the need for a team approach to treatment—doctors and nurses, that is, but also social workers, clergy, family, insurers, the surrounding community, and others.

Third, the study found a direct association between patients' contented acceptance of their situation and the quality of communication with their doctor. The more a doctor paid attention, the better patients felt. If, as earlier data shows, the problem with advance directives boils down to physicians' not listening, then the opportunity for a person to have calm final days depends largely on accomplishing the reverse. It is time to talk.

ONE STUDY IN WASHINGTON STATE approached end-of-life communication from both directions. Researchers asked both terminally ill patients and their doctors what barriers there were to meaningful talk.

Both sides came up with dozens of issues. Patients said they weren't ready to talk, they weren't that sick yet, they would rather concentrate on staying alive, they felt that talking about death could bring it closer, they worried that it would be too depressing for their doctor. Doctors said discussing end-of-life care takes extensive preparation, they had too little time to discuss these matters, they were not ready to give up on an aggressive approach to the illness, the patient wasn't sick enough yet.

In all, the findings are discouraging. Better communication equals better care, yet everyone had a large supply of reasons not to talk.

Then researchers asked what basis there might be for better communication. Patients said they were concerned about what would happen when they grew sicker, they trusted their doctor, they worried about being a burden on friends and family, they knew their doctor cared about them. Likewise, physicians said patients trusted them, they had cared for many other terminal patients, they worked in a system that expected them to have end-of-life-care-planning conversations.

In other words, there are as many aids to communication as there are barriers. The challenge is to overcome aversions so good work can be done.

"Access to palliative care is often delayed for dying, critically ill patients, because it is difficult for providers to articulate, and for patients and families to accept, that advanced supporting technology has been ineffective or will not result in a functional outcome that is acceptable to the patient." So conclude Harvard Medical School researchers working at Brigham and Women's Hospital in Boston.

"It is not humane to continue burdensome technology when there is no reasonable hope that it will be effective," their report continues. "The intravascular lines, support tubes and restraints used in this process are inherently uncomfortable and are associated with reduced mobility, autonomy and ability to communicate. When advanced support is associated with healing and the return of function, these discomforts are almost universally acceptable, but they are difficult to justify for patients who die."

The researchers thus decided to try an experiment: See if intensive communication makes patients' experience measurably better.

Under the plan, patients, their families, and the medical team met within three days of the patient's admission to the ICU. The meeting included reviewing the medical facts and options; discussing the patient's perspective on dying, dependence, and the discomforts of critical care; writing a care plan; and establishing clinical milestones—including time frames—against which the plan's performance could be measured.

Such meetings are a stark contrast with normal ICU care, in which patient goals are rarely if ever discussed, the care team communicates by reading each other's notes on the medical chart, patient and family education is haphazard, and the definition of success is a moving target.

The Boston experiment involved ongoing meetings to assess patients' progress, prepare for home or chronic care, and consider palliative care for patients not moving toward recovery. The study also measured what it called "non-consensus days"—the number of days in which the family, doctors, or nurses disagreed about what ought to be done.

The results were remarkable. The median length of patients' ICU stays fell 25 percent. Fewer patients entered intensive care at all, and the ICU was 6 percent less occupied. Not only did this save money, it enabled other admissions to the ICU, thereby affecting mortality beyond the study group.

The research also found that people agreed more often about what was best for the patient. Non-consensus days within families fell 91 percent. Non-consensus days within clinical teams dropped 94 percent. Imagine the time saved and heartache avoided through this harmony. Imagine end-of-life care without conflict.

The most striking finding: "One of our concerns about this intervention was that it might increase mortality rates, by introducing a bias toward palliative care when continued advance support technology would have preserved life. [Instead] the intensive communication intervention did not increase mortality. Rather there was a decrease in unadjusted overall mortality and a trend toward reduced mortality during the ICU stay."

Remember, this experiment was not about clinical care, but about communication. Families and doctors fought less, ICU use dropped, and patient mortality decreased.

If the goal is to replicate this experiment's gains through intensive communication, it will take practice. It will also require a change in culture that takes the heat out of the decisions.

"Routine discussions about end-of-life issues may serve all seriously ill patients, even those with a reasonable chance of stabilization or recovery," writes Timothy Quill, M.D. "Normalizing the discussion allows patients to learn about their right to high quality pain and symptom management, and educates physicians about patients' values and goals."

If people want to have more control over the shape of the end of their lives, they will have to be the ones who make this normalization possible. That takes courage. But the earlier a patient asks a question, the farther away any result will occur—and thus the less threatening the doctor's answer will be. Physicians need to show more courage, too, Dr. Quill says:

"Physicians are reluctant or unable to tell patients that they are approaching the end of their lives," he writes. So doctors give an unreasonably sunny forecast, or they delay out of fear of quelling a patient's hopes. "Not only is this not necessarily the case," Quill writes, "but failure to provide appropriate information about palliative care and prognosis can contribute to unnecessary pain and suffering."

For example, there is the issue of what to do should a person's heart stop. This discussion may be a patient's first exposure to the idea of limiting his treatments in a manner that leads to death, and thus the mere question may be terrifying. A doctor's capacity to relay the facts may make deciding infinitely easier, Quill argues. "Patients are less likely to choose CPR once they learn of its lack of efficacy."

There is, in other words, a direct cause and effect that is both emotional and clinical. Informed patients do not agonize, they decide. They also focus not on the treatment, as a physician might, but on its likely outcome. They make an intuitive but informed decision, based on quality. Quill writes that the physician's responsibility for enabling this process has, as a fortunate side effect, the gratification of doing it well: "When physicians provide their patients with the honesty, expertise, advocacy, compassion and commitment they would want for themselves and their families, they provide the highest quality of medical care possible."

CHAPTER TWENTY-SIX

"WE CAN CELEBRATE"

The last wishes of a seriously ill person have little or nothing to do with death. They are about life, about heightened awareness of its preciousness, about expressing individuality in the pursuit of small joys, about how death is an instant and every moment preceding that instant is living in all its fullness.

No two people will have the same end-of-life experience. But the potential for more Americans to achieve a fulfilling completion to their days is greater than ever. The question is not about how one dies but about how one lives.

ONE SUNDAY IN 1919, Warren G. Harding went to church in Palm Beach, Florida. After the service people lined up to shake hands with the president-elect. Harding worked his way through the crowd, which included a nine-year-old boy from Pennsylvania on vacation with his mother.

"As Harding came down, she pushed me forward as mothers do, and he patted me on top of the head and said, 'Nice boy.'"

So remembers that lad, now a ripe ninety-three years old. Chalmers Roberts lives north of Washington, D.C., in a house he and his wife Lois bought fifty years ago. His eyes are clear and his posture erect, and though he moves slowly there is neither a tremor nor any struggle for balance. On a crystalline September day he leads a visitor to the living room, where plate-glass doors look out on a conserved stretch of the Potomac

River valley. As Chalmers lowers himself onto the couch, a pendant swings out on its chain around his neck. It is an alarm, he explains, to call for aid should his heart stop beating.

Given his medical condition, it could happen at any moment. Yet Chalmers says he is not sure he would press the button. He just published an article in *The Washington Post* that described his quandary.

"I could be dead when you read this," the essay began. "But I thought it might be worthwhile to put down my thoughts about how I decided to skip a lifesaving heart operation."

After years of managing congestive heart failure, Chalmers learned that the valve between his heart and his aorta—the blood conduit to the lower body—had become faulty. His doctor suggested open-heart surgery to replace the valve. Chalmers asked what would happen if he said no.

"One of two outcomes will follow," he writes, "and the chance of one is about the same as the chance of the second. One possibility is that my aortic valve explodes with a rush of blood filling my body, ending my life instantly. Or I would again suffer from shortness of breath. I would return to the hospital, and would die in perhaps a couple of weeks as the valve slowly failed."

Chalmers is eager to explain why the surgery presented a genuine dilemma. "I grew up in the twentieth century, the most incredible in medical history. I have been the beneficiary. It always seemed to me that doctors were trained to extend life, and that's not the way I look at it at ninety-three. I think it ought to be about what kind of life you are extending."

Certainly he has led an exciting life, with decades as a top reporter at *The Washington Post* providing him with a front-row seat to history. Chalmers started at the newspaper in 1933, covering presidential press conferences on a salary of fifteen dollars a week. "I could just about live on it," he said. "I had three sets of clothes: good, bad, and terrible."

In the spring of 1941 he met Lois Hall. "April second, it was love at first sight," he recalls. It also was love in a hurry. They married that September.

Chalmers spent the war as a translator in the office that worked to break Japanese codes. His mission took him to Nagasaki not long after an atomic bomb had leveled the city.

"I was on a destroyer. I knew nothing about fallout. We went there in total curiosity. We just saw disaster." He sighs. "The thing I remember at Nagasaki was that the fire engines never got out of the firehouse."

After the war Chalmers covered Presidents Eisenhower, Kennedy, Johnson, Nixon, Ford, and Carter. His favorite person he ever met was Orville Wright. His favorite assignment was Nikita Khrushchev's visit to the United States. The living-room walls are covered with photos of Chalmers beside world leaders. His enduring views about life's value are shaped less by his news work and the war, though, than by two personal experiences.

One was watching a fellow newsman's wife die of Lou Gehrig's disease. "She ran an antiques store in Georgetown. She had to give it up, of course. The disease went on so slowly, and so relentlessly. Lois and I used to go and see her. The last time we saw her she was just curled up. She had a thing in her mouth, a kind of hose, that connected to this machine that could speak. I just thought it was the most miserable existence I've ever seen."

The other pivotal moment involved his father.

"My uncle was a wonderful man, and he called me up on the telephone. It was 1943. He said, 'Your dad's in the West Pennsylvania Hospital, and he is having a heart attack right now. Right now.' I just stayed on the line. He kept talking, reporting the situation to me. 'It's going badly. . . . He is dying. . . . He's dead.' All right there on the phone."

Chalmers's mother was on vacation with her sister. He could track her down immediately. Or he could wait a few days, until she arrived in Washington to visit Chalmers on her way home. He decided to wait.

"Well. She arrived at Union Station. I had the car parked there. Lois and I met these two ladies and took them out to the car. I put my mother in the front seat with me. I walked around the front of the car. I walked slowly. I got in. I gripped the steering wheel. And then I told her."

The memory makes him weep. "It is hard. It is hard to tell your mother her husband has died. It is very hard."

Why would a man whose sense of life's value remains that acute welcome death? This person is not depressed or despairingly sick. So, why?

Chalmers gives two reasons. The first is about lost love.

"We celebrated our sixtieth wedding anniversary on September eleventh, 2001—*that* September eleventh. She had been diagnosed with dementia before that, but physically she was pretty good. She'd broken a hip, and that changed our lifestyle. We had help during the day, and she had a walker. Then she was in the hospital with asthma. She was only really sick for a couple of weeks. She died that November third.

"If you're married you have certain pillow talks with your wife.

When you lose your wife of sixty years, you're reduced to sort of talking to yourself."

Chalmers takes off his glasses. "I began, after my wife died, thinking about life without her, and the status of my children and their children and where I went from here. I thought about that before going to sleep each night for some time. When the doctor sprang this operation idea on me, it sharpened the point."

Or, as his essay said, "I thought through as best I could the suggested heart operation, the long rehabilitation—and all to come home to what? A house with no spouse."

The other argument against surgery was recent medical experience.

"I learned a lot the last time I was in the hospital. I got really pissed off at all the poking and prodding. One day they took me downstairs where they have all their equipment. They ran me through three different tests, with different people. Then I was parked in the hallway, waiting for the guy to push me to the elevator and back to my room. Well, he didn't show up. I finally stopped some woman going by and said, 'Can you help me? I've been abandoned here.' She went next door. Then a guy came out and apologized and said they're running late today. Well. That was about when the doctor told me about the cardiac problem, and the surgery. It's something to do with age and dignity I guess—I said, 'Why do I want to do that?'"

Accepting that his existence will end does not mean that Chalmers is making light of his remaining time. On the contrary, he says, knowing life is finite makes it immeasurably richer. A good day includes a vigorous swim in the backyard pool. It involves a keen appreciation for the seasons passing outside those plate-glass doors. It surrenders nothing in being informed about current events and politics. It permits informed conversation on issues as varied as the history of the federal judiciary, the challenges facing post–Cold War Russia, and the next U.S. presidential election.

For now, too, Chalmers's life is about letters—hundreds of them stacked on the coffee table and couch, responses to his *Post* essay from all over the country. He is endeavoring to answer them, one by one.

"A lot are from widows whose husbands had some kind of operation in their eighties or nineties, and how badly it had turned out for the man. It made me realize that medicine, as great as it is, has its limits."

So does the control people have over their medical care, he says. "I've signed all sorts of papers that say don't put tubes in me, but the problem is that most doctors ignore that because they're afraid of being sued. It's ironic, if you think of my age. . . . In fact, I've decided if I make it into my ninety-fifth year, I'm going to have a big party. Here on the lawn. I will have over all of my doctors. We can celebrate."

The health system needs to change, Chalmers believes. People need to know that their experiences with gradual dying are not unique. Government policies must evolve to reflect the new realities. Medical education must adapt to the kind of care people need now. Health consumers must advocate for themselves better. It will take a "cultural transformation," he asserts.

This book's remaining chapters explore these ideas and others, accepting his challenge to find a better way for Americans' lives to close.

Some people may dismiss Chalmers's decision not to have surgery as less than heroic. After all, ninety-three years is a good long life. But that does not mean that Chalmers Roberts has any fewer tasks and ideas and loved ones to live for, nor any lighter attachment to the things of this world, nor diminished desire for new experiences, nor less curiosity about life's mysteries. This drive is human nature, he says. It is all a matter of *how* one lives, of the meaning each person gives to his or her finite time on earth. And how much control one has, or ought to have, as that time draws to a close.

Chalmers breaks his reverie with an apology: The afternoon is waning and he has work to do, reading and writing and all those letters to answer. He rises from his seat and guides a visitor to the front door. In the hall he pauses to gesture at a vase of flowers on the dining-room table, a dozen long-stemmed yellow roses.

"Aren't they beautiful?" he asks. Then, as firmly as if deciding something, he marches over to them. Chalmers spreads both palms on the table for balance. He leans down slowly, lowering himself until his face nearly touches the petals. He takes a long, strong sniff.

PART SIX

A GIFT OF SILVER

In Northern Darkness there lives a fish called K'un. This K'un is so huge that it stretches who knows how many thousand miles. When it changes into a bird it is called P'eng. This P'eng has a back spreading who knows how many thousand miles. And when it thunders up into flight, its wings are like clouds hung clear across the sky. It churns up the sea and sets out on its migration to Southern Darkness. . . .

P'eng beats the water for three thousand miles, whirling up vast gale storms, then climbs ninety thousand miles on the winds. It flies on and on for six months, and then it rests.

Heat waves shimmering, dust and ash and everything alive all buffeted among one another in air—and then it rests.

—CHUANG-TZU

CHAPTER TWENTY-SEVEN

LOBSTER NEWBURG

I have some scary news."

It was my sister Amy on the phone. I was standing at the front desk of the old inn in Ripton, Vermont, at the Breadloaf Writers' Conference. It was August 1988 and I was there between semesters of graduate school, working as a member of the social staff. The morning lectures had just ended, and writers from all over the country were banging in and out the screen door right beside the phone. I could not have had less privacy if I'd been standing on the Little Theater stage during a poetry reading.

"Let me guess," I joked. "You're pregnant."

"Dad has an aneurysm," she said. "Of his abdominal aorta. And it ruptured. He's in surgery right now."

That was how it began, my education in human mortality. At the age of twenty-eight, I'd lost loved ones before: grandparents, an uncle, even a beloved friend six weeks after his twenty-seventh birthday. But those deaths had all happened elsewhere, away from me. For those people my role was to receive the news, nothing more. I was not a participant, not a witness. In my father's case, though, scary news was just the beginning.

How unprepared was I for what lay ahead? Well, I did not even know whether I should leave Breadloaf. My friend Carol Knauss, nominally the conference's secretary but in practical terms its administrative maestro, told me to go at once. Ben Reynolds, my boss on the staff, declared that he would not permit me to stay. Besides, he added with an arm thrown around my shoulders, I could always come back. I tossed clothes and guitar into my car, hugged friends, and drove over the winding pass to Hancock and points south.

Who was this man I was praying for while I drove? He was born in Albany, New York, and aside from attending college in Massachusetts and serving in the Pacific theater in World War II, that was where he had always lived. He followed his curmudgeonly father in the family insurance business, until he realized he could not afford to educate his growing family on that income. My father sold the company to its employees, went to work for a small Albany bank, and over fifteen years built it into a regional holding company with assets of about $20 billion. He accomplished all of this by dint of a sharp mind and a strong back. He also believed success came to people with integrity and character, so he lived a muscularly virtuous life. He went to church. He did not drink. His only vices were chocolate and tobacco, both indulged in excessively. Otherwise, he kept himself shaved and clean, dressed sharply, and rarely even swore. For lazy people and fools, he developed an unconscious dismissive gesture, a sweeping away with the back of his hand. His standards of conduct for his children were high, but for himself were higher. He was as unbending as hickory.

That August my father was vacationing on Cape Cod with my mother. The weekend before his illness the entire family—at that time numbering seven children, four spouses, and six grandkids—had gathered for his sixty-fifth birthday. He loved it, especially his time with the grandchildren. My father had been in great spirits all weekend, except for an odd foreshadowing period Saturday night when for some mysterious reason he could not stop sweating.

Then, and a brief episode the following morning—just the two of us strolling in the driveway—in which he criticized me yet again for my insufficiently promising career prospects, as well as for my persistence in dating a woman he maintained was of the wrong religion. The conversation ended with him walking away, making that dismissive hand gesture while snorting over his shoulder, "I am not proud of you."

I left that evening. Five afternoons later he had felt dizzy, then exhausted. At midnight, on his way to the bathroom, he collapsed. My mother called an ambulance while he protested that he was fine. At that time Cape Cod had two hospitals within striking distance of my folks' place. Had my father gone to Hyannis that night, there would have been no operating room for emergency vascular surgery. Minutes after his body's main blood vessel sprang its leak, he would simply have died. But for some reason he chose Falmouth, with a small medical center in a postcard-pretty town that had both an OR and a surgeon standing by. The doctor told my father his aorta was leaking and required emergency surgery. My father asked if there was time for him to step outside and smoke a cigarette. The surgeon laughed and said some pain medicine might be more in order. My father said no thanks, but a few seconds later winced and said he might take some of that pain stuff after all. In surgery, just as the doctor was opening him up, the aorta ruptured. My father's heart pumped its blood supply out on the operating table. The surgeon clamped off the bleeding and set about making repairs. It took all night. Although my father required a transfusion of seventeen units of blood, at least he had not died. Not entirely.

The central question, as our family assembled from around the country, was whether he would pee. My brother Mike, a medical student in St. Louis, explained that half of aneurysm rupture victims die before reaching the hospital, half of the rest die in surgery, half of the remainder die in the following forty-eight hours, and the fundamental factor in the survival of that remaining one-eighth is whether their kidney function returns.

My father's trickled, two days after surgery, then stopped. The staff at that little hospital was astonishingly patient with the gang of us, plus friends, clergy, my father's colleagues. We gathered. We waited. We prayed.

One morning we had a call from the local harbormaster, asking us to please come move my father's sailboat. We had all chipped in to buy him a well-used twenty-seven-foot O'Day the year before, for his sixty-fourth birthday. Apparently he'd gone out for an hour's calm motoring on the afternoon before he became ill. Afterward, instead of mooring the boat properly, he had parked it at the main dock. It was blocking everyone. For my father, a man fastidious in propriety, it was an inexplicable breach. My brothers Pete and John went with me to the small marina. We clambered aboard, and there on the seat was the floating lanyard to which the boat's key was normally attached. But the key was broken, snapped in half with the rest still in the ignition. It was another sign that my father had been ill hours before he knew it.

We were just untying from the pier, planning to paddle to the mooring, when my brother Greg came careening in my car down the ramp. "He's fading fast," Greg yelled to us. "He's dying right now."

Pete retied the boat in its improper spot. I drove. My car was a Honda Civic, weighing perhaps fifteen hundred pounds and now carrying four two-hundred-pound men in a flat panic. That day was also the annual running of the Falmouth Road Race, which draws thousands of athletes from around New England. The race follows Route 28, which is also the most direct way to the hospital, and there were runners all along the road. A mediocre driver, I honked, I shouted, I swerved. As they leapt out of my path the runners and race volunteers looked at me less with dismay than with puzzlement. What kind of an idiot could this be? I know I damaged my little car's engine and clutch, and to this day remain amazed that I didn't hit anyone.

This all happened before cell phones became common, so there was no way of knowing what we would find at the hospital. We screeched to a halt and ran in, sprinting to the tiny intensive-care unit.

Our hurry was for naught. He had bounced back. His pulse was steady. His blood pressure, bolstered by huge doses of dopamine, had recovered. We celebrated in the corridor; we made fists and danced around.

In retrospect, I realize that the car was not all that was careening. At that moment, veering from panic without purpose to euphoria without justification, we were textbook cases of the American approach to death. We were completely unprepared, unschooled, and unassisted. Had my father died that morning, there would have been no concern about how much medical technology to use. Because he was dying slowly, though, no one ever questioned using every tool imaginable, not only hoping for a miracle but expecting one. Somehow, inexplicably, we forgot that everyone dies.

Yet I paused in the hallway gladness to take a good look at my father. The breathing tube kept his mouth open, so his lips had dried and cracked to the verge of bleeding. A drug to relax him so he would not fight the ventilator had left his eyes open too long; they were painfully red, the corners rimmed with pus. His hands were strapped down to thwart any reflexive attempt to remove his tubes. He had a rough beard, an anathema to my father's always polished appearance. And with his kidneys still not working, he was beginning to bloat.

My sisters, Casey and Amy, stood on either side of my mom. They took notes, they asked doctors questions for her, they offered an arm for support, they paid nonstop attention to her needs. We could not decide whether my mother should stand by my father's bed in case he awoke, or remain in the waiting room and be spared the sight of his suffering.

I was not a decision maker there, nor would any sixth child out of seven have that standing. No, I was a passenger, ballast, a spare set of hands for carrying a suitcase or dealing with the sailboat. I was a spectator.

Late that afternoon Greg and I realized that no one had eaten all day. We took it upon ourselves to find a deli and order a dozen sandwiches. We sat on a bench on the nearby village green to wait while the food was prepared. Greg sat so close that our shoulders rubbed. "Do you think he's going to die?" he asked me. "No," I said with a certainty that I genuinely felt. "He is too strong, and not that old, and too attached to his grandchildren." Greg replied that the real question was how much of himself our dad would lose from this. His foot jiggled ceaselessly as we spoke. Then he pressed the bottom of his shoe against the bottom of mine and we were silent a moment. No matter what, Greg said, things were never going to be the same.

On the way back to the deli, I was thinking about lobster Newburg. It was one of my father's favorite stories about his father, Peter Kiernan Sr., a notorious grouch who died before I was born. It seems that on his eighty-third birthday, the housekeeper/cook/nurse who took care of Peter Sr. came in to wake him in the morning. She wished him a happy birthday. He replied gruffly that he was being joined for birthday lunch by three gentlemen friends, and he wished her to serve them lobster Newburg. "In that case," she said, "I'll need to go to the store. We'll need sherry, cheese, butter, cream, and of course lobsters." "Make it rich," the old curmudgeon told her, "nice and thick."

When lunchtime arrived, she had set the table for four and was ready to serve the meal. But no gentlemen friends had come. My grandfather sat at the table alone. "Don't worry about them," he said, "I'll go ahead." She brought in the tureen of lobster Newburg. Peter Sr. proceeded to serve himself plate after heaping plate. When the housekeeper came later to clear the table, she found him unconscious. She called my father, who called the doctor, who called an ambulance. They took Peter Sr. to the hospital, pumped his stomach, and kept him overnight.

The next day he returned home and went to bed early. In the morning the housekeeper welcomed my grandfather home, and asked if there was something gentle and restorative she might make him for lunch that day. "I know just the thing," he answered, holding one finger aloft: "lobster Newburg."

The woman blanched, went to the kitchen, and immediately called my father. He rang up the doctor again, explained the situation, and asked what he should do. The doctor's reply was my father's favorite part of the story. He said, "If he wants lobster Newburg, for God's sake, give it to him. If he needs his stomach pumped again, we'll pump his stomach again.

He's eighty-three years old. How many more times will he get to eat his favorite dish?"

Greg and I carried bags of soda and chips and sandwiches into the small waiting room, and everyone immediately set to eating. I just grabbed a cup of ginger ale and went down the hall to look at Dad. He lay there inert. The machinery was so unfamiliar and unnatural, it was hard to believe it was keeping him alive. I suppose many sons see their father as a powerful figure; for all that mine intimidated me, it felt off-kilter for him to be so passive, so little an agent of his destiny. They had put a strange mattress under him—it looked like a foam egg carton—and I suppose they were guarding against potential bedsores. I stood there, trying to imagine what would be the equivalent of lobster Newburg for a man in this predicament. All of a sudden his eyes fluttered. Then they opened wide. I ran to the hallway and called my mother, who came at top speed.

She looked into his sore eyes. She stroked his hair. She told him that he was getting great care and everyone was taking good care of her, too. She told him quietly that she loved him. He tried to answer, and she told him to hush. He ran a dry tongue over his now ravaged lips. My mother turned and dipped her fingertips in my ginger ale. Then she touched them to his lips, and his tongue came out for a taste. "Dear God," she said, "he likes it."

His eyes closed. She told him to sleep, to rest, to concentrate his energy on getting better. My father lapsed back into his coma. It was the last time his eyes opened in this world. And I wondered: What is the difference between lobster Newburg and ginger ale?

HIS KIDNEYS FAILED. He ran a fever, sign of an infection somewhere. Days passed with no flicker of consciousness. My father needed dialysis. The earnest doctors of Falmouth said there was no more they could do. We had reached one of many opportunities in which we could have set a limit, acknowledged what had happened, and accepted what was certain to occur.

Instead, we demanded more care, more interventions, more heroism. We pushed for my father to be transported to Massachusetts General Hospital. Informed that he would not survive the trip by ambulance, we advocated, cajoled, and insisted—and the next day loaded him onto a medical helicopter that swooped him away north to Boston. Standing on the ground as the rotor wash threw sand in my face, squinting as the giant dragonfly lifted away, I felt the drama of it all. But I also wondered why we were doing this. Who was it for? What was the goal? How much of my questioning had to do with unresolved conflict between my father and me? We were taking him to the best hospital around, but was that the best idea?

Mass General is a huge complex of buildings, labs, and garages. The first time I entered the front doors, it took me twenty minutes to find my father. That night Mike and I moved in with our cousins Ann and Rob, who showed saintly patience with our comings and goings over the following weeks. My mother and sisters shared a hotel room, while my other brothers took turns bunking with friends and going home to their families. Everything else in our lives—jobs, children, education—we put on hold.

Instead, we became an ICU family. We met with doctors, or tried to. We followed my father's treatment, or tried to. We watched him balloon with fluids, so that he no longer looked like the man we knew. We ignored the cost, knowing his health insurance would cover most of the care and we would somehow find a way, later on, to swing the rest. My sisters continued playing goalie between the world and my mother, whose primary emotional expression was white-lipped rage. The days accumulated, and my father's ICU beard grew. Finally Mike filched a clean bedpan, filled it with water, and snuck in at night to shave him.

There were other ways of giving love, for each of us. My mother prayed with him several times daily. Pete read him the newspaper's business section. Casey massaged his arms. I told him about the world outside, the coming of fall, what I had seen on my walks to and from the hospital. I wanted to sit on the bed for these talks, but the rails were locked in a raised position, so I contented myself with laying one hand on his upper arm.

Meanwhile, my father continued to need huge helpings of dopamine, which maintained an acceptable blood pressure but caused potassium to accumulate in dangerous quantities in his blood. Every other day he would undergo dialysis, to scrub the potassium out. Each dialysis treatment would improve his color but reduce his blood pressure. The solution was always more dopamine, thus more potassium, and so on.

No one ever used the words *pointless* or *vicious cycle* or even *futile*. We just soldiered on, chatting with false optimism at my father's bedside in case he could hear, standing by for anything my mother might need, trying to find a role for ourselves when there was so little we could do, endeavoring to convince the diligent ICU staff that this man was special, was someone who deserved to heal and live and rise from that bed.

There was one day of hope, or so we thought. That morning I heard my father's dopamine level was down to 9,000 units, after the previous day's 10,000 and a prior high of 12,500. "Isn't that great news?" I said to Mike. He said no. A heart attack victim typically gets five or ten units. Dad was still thousands away from "great news."

That afternoon one of the doctors delivered half of the information we needed to hear. In a waiting room that was temporarily home to two other families besides ours, he told us that my father would never recover to what we had known. He would need dialysis for the rest of his life. He would have to use a wheelchair. His brain function would be permanently impaired. His memory, communication, and motor skills would be diminished. He would need round-the-clock nursing. And that was all presuming that he somehow bounced back again, miraculously, and awoke from his coma.

I went into my father's room. A salve had healed his eyes. A tracheotomy tube allowed him to breathe through his throat, so his mouth was healing. But he was so big now, swelling toward three hundred pounds. His neck was like a tire. His hands, in their restraints, were beefy with fluid. Only his ear—the poor misshapen ear he had wounded in the war—looked as it should. If it was painful for me to see him this way, I thought, what agony it must be for him to live in that swollen skin. If he was aware of it, that is.

That night Pete, Greg, and I took a meandering walk around Back Bay, the handsome neighborhood built in the early 1800s. We found a pub and went in for a beer. The waitress thought we'd come for dinner. She brought menus and recited the specials. That night's featured entree: lobster Newburg.

It was like a kick in the belly. But the coincidence also gave me the courage I needed. As soon as the waitress delivered the beers, I told my brothers I was thinking about leaving. There was nothing I could do to help. I was imposing on my cousins. I was missing the semester. I could return on a moment's notice. I did not add that I could not bear to see my father tortured any longer. I just said maybe it was time I went back to Iowa.

Their reactions surprised me. "There's nothing for you to do here, buddy," Greg said. Pete agreed. "Dad would want you to be doing your job," he said.

The next morning my mother not only echoed their advice, she urged me to go. "The things you see here will stick with you, in your memory," she said. "You should remember your father alive and well instead."

It was too late to make that happen. He had been comatose for twenty-one days, and the images of those weeks are indelible—eclipsing his living memory for years to come. Still, we agreed I would return to Boston in three weeks. Inside, I vacillated between doubting that I could hold out longer than a few days and questioning whether I would ever come back at all.

It was not a lack of love for my father, I believed then and maintain today. In fact, it was that I did love him and could not remain a powerless witness to his suffering any longer.

That afternoon we had our good-bye. We were alone: me, my father, the machines. His last words to me, about not being proud, now had a frightening resonance. In many ways he was already gone. My father, a patriarch never lacking for will or wit, lay absent in every way but body.

I was nervous. I felt an entirely new sadness, like a clenched fist where my heart ought to be. I tried to lower the railing but couldn't get it to release. So I reached over the bar and laid my palms on his chest.

"Let us end this," I told him, my words coming out formally for reasons I still do not understand. "Let us cease our struggles and acknowledge the love and respect we have for each other. Old man, let us put down our arguments at last. I honor you and all you have done for me." I began to cry, tears falling on his thin hospital bedshirt. "I can barely speak but I must say that I am filled with gratitude to you."

His face did not flicker. The machinery wheezed and sighed.

That night I drove to Albany, the next day to Iowa City. I attended classes, did my homework, and went without sleep. Because I was in two places, I was in neither place. Every day I called back East twice, morning and evening. The news was never good.

Finally even Mass General's doctors felt compelled to deliver the second half of the truth they had begun a week before. The dopamine-dialysis cycle was going nowhere. My father was not getting better. The person we knew and loved was gone, and it was time to let his body go as well. If we ceased dialysis, the potassium would painlessly put him to sleep.

There were eight people to decide: some on the scene, some by phone. Some were pragmatic; others began mourning. Greg argued that we were giving up too soon. We had no idea that our situation was commonplace. All of us felt the absence of our usual decision maker.

Finally we agreed to stop dialysis. The doctors said it would mean that only a few days remained. But there was an error in the medical orders, and my father received the blood-cleansing treatment again anyway. The gray area we had entered became even murkier. The next time his dialysis came due, a Tuesday, he remained in his ICU room. Fifteen hundred miles away, I held my breath. But not for long.

My father died on a Thursday, at about ten P.M. My mother and three of my siblings were present. She phoned me in Iowa to say it had happened quietly, without struggle. Since my sister's initial call about something scary, twenty-eight days had passed. There had been no redemption, nothing saved.

The demanding workaday world, gone utterly away for that month, returned with all of its trivial demands the moment my father left it. In addition to grieving his death, I had to reckon with all our unresolved issues. I would have to do it alone. The task would take years.

My mother gave the sailboat away the following summer, to a Cape Cod high school. But I still have that lanyard, the one with the broken key.

Peter D. Kiernan Jr. was a decent, generous, bright, hardworking, moral, intelligent man. He had educated me, fed me, supported me, and disapproved of me. When we arrived at the church for his funeral, the matter of the casket was like so many occasions before: The sixth child does not stand at the fore, of course. I remembered decades earlier when we put up a basketball hoop. While my brothers sawed and nailed and measured, my only task was to hold. Likewise the unwritten rules of birth order are in effect even at a funeral. As we assembled at the foot of the steep church steps, two of my brothers held a brass handle on each side of the casket, while I took my position at its heel. My sisters inched ahead, supporting my mother. A bagpiper stood in the church's nave playing "Going Home."

But then I received a small yet meaningful gift. As we climbed the steps to the door, the weight of the casket tilted toward my end, and the burden of my father slid from my brothers down to me. It was heavy, the oaken coffin with his bloated body within. Once again it was my task to hold. It took some effort to keep my father level. But I managed. And I felt supremely glad for my arms and my strength—and for the opportunity, just for that moment, to bear him.

CHAPTER TWENTY-EIGHT

A BOWL OF APPLESAUCE

S eptember again, but four years later, my mother found a lump in her breast. I was about to travel to Greece with a buddy on a long-planned vacation that she encouraged me to take. Recently she had remarried, a widower named Bob Callahan who lost his first wife to breast cancer. With Bob at her side, she urged me to go ahead. I protested, saying I would not enjoy myself while worrying about her, but she dismissed it. Whatever her situation, she insisted, life had to go on.

That was Mary Agnes Kiernan's philosophy. My mother had no college education, yet insisted that each of her children become impeccably educated. Struck by multiple sclerosis when her brood ranged in age from four to fourteen, she overcame a resulting bout of depression and not only walked again but marched right back into parenting, work, travel, charitable boards, and a central role in my father's career success. She made lists of tasks and took pointed pleasure in crossing each item off, as if its actual accomplishment was less important than the fact that it had succumbed to her determination and organization. The central force behind her recovery—and her subsequent life's successes—was simple: unyielding, mulish, Irish stubbornness. She was loyal to friends and savage to people who crossed her. If anyone told my mother something bad that one of her children had done, she would insist with spitting rage that it could not possibly be true, then come home and discipline the offender with identical vigor. Her saving graces, fortunately, were a surpassing sense of humor and a love of children that was as fierce as her temper.

I called from Athens and learned that it was definitely cancer. At Santorini I learned it was present in several lymph nodes, so the disease had likely spread. By Rhodes they had found it in her throat. On Kalymnos, over a 1940s vintage phone so frustratingly scratchy that I nearly smashed it against the wall, I learned that she would undergo a lumpectomy and lymph-node removal, followed by chemotherapy. My buddy was sympathetic about how joyless the vacation had become. When I stopped in New York on the way home, my mother was livid that I had gone on the trip. For my part, I was angry that she had insisted I go, and angrier that she had forgotten her urging. It took weeks for us to return to good standing with each other, which we accomplished only by admitting a difficult truth: Neither of us had expected the situation to be anywhere near so bad. And when doctors took an X-ray of her chest before the lumpectomy, they discovered a mass in her lung. She was in serious trouble.

If the chemo was hard on her, my mother never showed it. She scheduled her organized life around the biweekly treatments, she wore her wig, and she went to church with her usual frequency. Bob developed a careworn look that would haunt his expression for the next thirteen months.

It was not a time of stasis for my mother, though. She continued her charity work. She made plans for a family wedding. She spoke about going to Rome, her favorite city, and seeing Switzerland with Bob. Granted, her energy flagged easily. She lost some of her life's pleasures, too. For instance, each evening since her twenties she had enjoyed a bourbon on the rocks—a single drink before dinner even in the mayhem years of raising seven young children, even when she had five teenagers at once. But the chemo changed her sense of taste. One night that winter when I served her a bourbon, she took one sip and said, "Damn it. I can't even enjoy a good drink anymore."

The irony, despite her unremitting bad news, was that it was also a time of great love. My mother had taken the loss of my father hard; she was angry and adrift. But the summer after he died, when she went alone to the Cape, I happened to land a teaching job just north of Boston. Several nights a week I drove down to help with chores, take her out to dinner, even be her date at parties when she took her first tentative steps back into socializing.

That summer we built a friendship beyond any we'd had when my father was alive. She confided in me when she began to have feelings for Bob. I called her very early on when, after a long time on my own, I met a lovely woman named Amy. She asked my opinion one time when Bob had taken her for granted. I confided in her that things with Amy had become

serious quickly. She invited me to visit only days before her planned but
secret elopement with Bob, and I threw them a three-person engagement
party. As her dire health situation became clear, I saw an obvious symmetry; in a pause between my mother's chemo treatments, I asked Amy to
marry me. She said yes.

Instantly my mother had a focus. It was her kind of challenge, an opportunity to be determined and organized. There was no way she would
not make her part of the wedding weekend thoughtful and elegant. There
was no chance that she would die without completing the job of seeing
me wed. Amy and I chose a date in mid-September 1993, just after her
chemo would wrap up, with a little cushion for her to regain strength.

My mother had a difficult summer, losing weight, losing stamina. But
she chose a dress, sent invitations to the Friday night party, gave everyone
instructions to keep the days orderly. My mother had something to live for.

She also went to a surgeon, a renowned thoracic specialist at Memorial Sloan-Kettering in New York City—one of the top cancer hospitals in
the country. He reviewed her case, read her charts, saw the cancer in her
throat and lung, and then proposed a hemiquadrantectomy. In this surgery, the physician makes an incision that begins just under the ear,
sweeps down the chest, then reverses direction to end below the armpit.
Everything on that side—the lung, the throat, the entire arm—is removed.
Everything. Gone. He said it was her "only hope for a cure."

My mother called Mike, by that time a third-year resident. Mike swallowed his anger and explained. She had what is called a small-cell cancer,
a kind that cannot be cut out of a body. In fact, doctors often tell small-
cell cancer patients that the one good thing about their illness is that they
will not face a battery of surgeries. In this case, the doctor had proposed a
procedure that would be profoundly disfiguring and excruciatingly painful, would require that she receive help in all kinds of everyday functions
for the rest of her life (buttoning a shirt, going to the bathroom)—and in
the end her survival would not be extended by a single day.

We can only wonder what happens to patients without a medical resident son they can call for advice. The extremity of the doctor's idea not
only caused my mother to reject the surgery but also formed her thinking
for the rest of the illness. This was not going to be about chasing miracles.
It was going to be about dying on her terms. It was going to be about control. For a woman who prized organization and determination, this was
her turf.

The wedding weekend arrived, and my mother was magnificent. Bob could barely speak, he was so worried. But my mother made champagne toasts, threw a great party, gave a reading during the ceremony, danced with me at the reception. Midway through the evening she gave me a fierce hug. She wished Amy and me every blessing, but she was heading to her room. She was exhausted. "Now that I'm going," she said, patting my cheek, "you children can go ahead and behave shamefully."

And we did. I don't remember a time when my brothers and sisters partied with greater abandon. A piece of it was celebrating the wedding and Stephen finally settling down with a woman who seemed loving and decent. But there was also a sense of last hurrah, of the end of our idea of "family" being not far away. We danced with flower arrangements on our heads. We staged bullfights with tablecloths and serving forks. We climbed on one another's shoulders and spun like tops. The band's lead singer, a bohemian screamer with wild hair and a saucy style, asked through the microphone, "What is with you people? You have gone entirely wild."

Immediately afterward, my mother began an accelerated decline. Four days after the vows, she had trouble breathing. A tumor in her throat was blocking the airway. She received emergency radiation to clear a passage, an excellent use of palliative care, but everyone knew the cancer was winning. Amy and I decided our honeymoon could wait. We traveled to New York to see her constantly, sometimes twice a week. To everyone's good fortune, Mike finished his residency and moved in as her primary caretaker.

All that October my mother remained busy. She rewrote her will to acknowledge that she might not outlast the year. When she learned how much of her estate would be lost to taxes, she began slipping me cash. She sent notes to friends. She had priests visit often. She consoled Bob. She planned her funeral, every detail set but the date of her death on the prayer card. She threw herself a birthday party, inviting the whole family.

That afternoon she noticed that her granddaughter Katelyn had been avoiding her. My mother called Katelyn over, pulling the eight-year-old onto her lap. They made a moment's small talk before my mother plunged in.

"You know, lambie, you don't have to be afraid about what's happening," she said. "I'm not afraid. You see, dying doesn't hurt."

Katelyn fiddled with her braid. "I know that." Then she held on tight.

We each had those moments, quiet and private, most of all Mike. Although I suspect she felt considerable embarrassment whenever he helped her go to the bathroom or lifted her out of the tub, it was a huge advantage for my mother to have a personal doctor. I can only guess at Mike's gratification from giving such help when it was so needed.

But the benefits went beyond the two of them. One day when I stood at the bedside, my mother asked me to help her turn over. This was late in the illness; she had not been out of bed in days. I scooped under her arm and ribs, hoisted, and immediately realized that the task was beyond me. Her muscle tone was gone. To use an unfortunate expression, she was dead weight. I tried again. All I did was stretch her arm. I struggled on, pushing her thigh now, but her grunts told me that I was only making her uncomfortable. Finally in a panic I called Mike from the next room. He came in, asked what was needed, and bent over the bed on the far side. There he grabbed the edge of a towel that lay beneath my mother. With a slow, steady draw, he pulled the towel upward. It slid under her, easing my mother gently onto her other side. Then he smoothed the towel flat, so he could turn her back again later. I admired Mike's competence, I envied his ability to care for her so correctly, and I loved him for what he was doing to make her dying easier.

My moment of quiet connection arrived in the form of applesauce. I had the privilege, one November afternoon very near the end, of spooning applesauce laced with medicine into my mother's mouth. She ate slowly, swallowing with effort, and I was careful not to hurry her or spill. It was as intimate a moment as we ever shared. I reminded her that my father in affectionate moments had called her "Mary Applesauce." I told her she was preparing me to feed my future children, should they come. That got her to smile between spoonfuls. I told her I thought her life was a triumph of will—raising seven children, guiding us through adolescence with no disasters, seeing each of us educated far beyond her schooling, watching us find our way in the world. I thanked her for heroic efforts during the wedding. Feeding my mother in small bites—to make it easy for her and to make it last for me—I told her I was grateful for the friendship we had developed during her early widowhood and was glad the bond had endured once her grieving eased. With a cloth I wiped her lips, and then my eyes.

She said, "Don't cry, lambie. You were always an easy baby."

Four days later, at her home, in her room, with her family and husband praying at her bedside, with her final sacrament accomplished by a soft-spoken priest, with her pain silenced by morphine, with a household calm not unlike the quiet around a sleeping infant, Mary Agnes Kiernan Callahan took a slow last breath and died. There was nothing left undone between us. There was nothing left undone in her life at all.

· · ·

ALTHOUGH THERE ARE AN INFINITE number of things to recount about my mother's life, there is one remaining point to make about her dying. It concerns a mistake.

She had made all the funeral arrangements, of course. My mother would be in a coffin she approved, at a funeral home she selected, for a closed-casket wake at hours she specified. Amy and I arrived ahead of time with Bob, to make sure everything was in order. The undertaker had made one error: Her casket was open.

It is always a shock to see someone you love lying dead. The absence of animating energy is so powerful, the stillness such a presence. Embalming and makeup notwithstanding, there is no ambiguity. This is an object utterly without life.

But not without meaning. Because once we absorbed the surprise, the three of us stood before her with reverence. The reason was her face, her expression. It was as tough and determined as in any stubborn moment of her living days. Her brow was firm. Her jaw was stuck straight forward.

I turned to Bob. "She looks like a woman in the process of winning an argument."

He laughed. "I know that look. We had all better behave today."

We called the attendant, who closed the casket before anyone else arrived. The wake was crowded and long, which is the best tribute to a life. Eventually the people thinned out and went home. We were all tired. But Greg asked if he could see my mother one last time. The attendant said of course, and I stood alongside while they opened the lid again.

Greg saw her face and said, "Wow."

"Pretty amazing, eh?" I replied.

"I know what she's saying." He chuckled. "Hey, Death, screw you."

SIX WEEKS LATER Amy and I received a shipment from a store in New York City. Inside the shipping box was a fancier box, and inside that one was a present, a complete place setting of our silver pattern. But that was not all. Also inside that fancy box was a note, wishing us a happy first married Christmas together, with much love—written in my mother's inimitable hand. It was a classic gesture. Sometime in late September before taking to her bed, my mother had done her Christmas shopping, written notes, arranged the shipping. I was touched by her thoughtfulness. But there was something bigger about it, too, something almost triumphant. I was uplifted by how completely—right to the very end, and now with this gift even beyond it—her bright character had remained undimmed.

CHAPTER TWENTY-NINE

ILLNESS AS OPPORTUNITY

There was a process, for me and my family, an education through these two deaths. We discovered that the manner of a death has meaning, reverberating long after the person has died. In my father's illness, I can instantly conjure feelings of helplessness at seeing his dignity stripped away, a sense of complicity in his suffering, a regret that our last conversation was a conflicted one.

My mother was right about those images, too. Even now I can picture his sore eyes in the Falmouth hospital, his cracked lips. I hope he never regained consciousness sufficiently to realize that his hands were strapped down. In all, I feel an anguish quite apart from the sense of loss. This was a powerful man who shaped so much of his life. Yet his dying did not go well. And no repair of that is possible.

By contrast, my mother's dying process was marked by rewards and accomplishments. Of course she did not achieve everything she hoped. There were places she wanted to travel, experiences she'd hoped to enjoy, a new marriage she'd embraced with full optimism that would see an early end. Of course, too, there was great sadness for us all when she died.

But the waning of her life occurred on her terms. She attended important occasions. She left things in order, which was important to her. She made preparations from the financial to the spiritual. She had a chance to exercise medical control, when offered the choice of that surgery. She relished that her final care was inexpensive. She made peace with her children and played one last matriarchal role for her grandchildren.

My mother also left an image that remains in my mind forever, but it is not one of weakness or powerlessness or defeat. It is as feisty as her determined Irish temper: In the end, her jaw was stuck straight out.

THERE IS A STARK CONTRAST between the old and new ways of reckoning with gradual dying: the frustrations of the former and the gratifications of the latter, the technology of the first and the human touch of the second, the expense of one and the emotional richness of the other.

Obviously the stories here provide only one of many possible versions of what happened. I'm sure each of my siblings has a different memory and a unique perspective on what my parents' dying processes signified. So may the doctors and nurses who provided care, the friends who supported us, the clergy who prayed with us.

Yet I suspect every version would agree on the strongest lessons: We learned how to help a loved one die well. We developed the metaphysical maturity to realize that death is something we can indeed bear to face, and should face—because if we do, we can shape its meaning and effect. We found a way to be loving during pain, and thereby reduce a person's suffering. We learned that we must shoulder the responsibility of our own death, to attain a fitting passage for ourselves. We realized that death is not an afterthought of life but an opportunity to reaffirm all of life that is noblest, most compassionate, most courageous.

It is attainable for many more Americans, too, but not without changes in law and policy, in medical training and hospital habits, and above all in the attitudes of patients and families who refuse to accept a dying process that is less than what they deserve.

What we learned in our family microcosm is precisely what American society needs to discover.

PART SEVEN

THE LESSON OF THE LEAVES

Lord let me die, but not die out.
—JAMES DICKEY

Be sure to live your life,
because you are a long time dead.
—SCOTTISH PROVERB

CHAPTER THIRTY

THE ENDLESS CYCLE

I n Northern Vermont where I live, the winters are long and sometimes Arctic cold. The months beforehand are called "stick season" because leafless forests stand bare and gray. Dark comes early. Once winter wanes, instead of the spring that offers colorful release in most places, we have "mud season" because of the sodden bogs the state's primarily dirt roads become. Plants are slow to bud; frost surrenders its deep grip reluctantly. When summer finally arrives, it is clear-skied paradise, the air seemingly energized and the days long and bright. But that season flies; lovely Lake Champlain is comfortable swimming only about nine weeks a year.

In all, it is a harsh climate. And yet every year there is one time, one beautiful blessed time, when there is no lovelier place on earth. It is magnetic, too. From all across the planet, people are drawn to learn the lesson of the leaves.

Of course, the departure of green foreshadows our own mortality. Of course, the withering and falling leaves bring on a sweet melancholy. Of course, the precision of stars on clear October nights emphasizes the infinite, before which we are so miniscule and brief.

But the leaves speak powerfully against these messages. As they die, they incandesce. From a biological standpoint they are simply drying up, revealing pigments that had been concealed by the chemistry of photosynthesis. But that perspective only reveals the limitations of scientific description. What the heart understands is that the woods become stunning: birches turning graceful yellow, sugar maples a fiery orange, oaks a somber brown, sumac a red so bright it's almost a sound.

That is the lesson of the leaves: that life as it wanes can be distilled into its purest shape and that this final form can be more beautiful than all the days beforehand. This is the instruction that nature gives us.

American culture today prizes youth and vigor, in contrast with societies that revere age and wisdom. But now baby boomers themselves are aging. They have always been a colorful tribe, challenging conventions and defining new norms. Perhaps this group's focus will shift as their hair grays and they suffer the loss of their parents and a few friends. Perhaps they will recognize the potential for brilliance and brightness in their lives' final days—and find themselves moved to enact changes in the law to nurture that opportunity, to demand new policies that reflect the winter not so far ahead, to advocate for themselves and their loved ones so that their experience is not like a woodlot clear-cut for timber, but like a forest repeating an endless and mysterious annual cycle.

Perhaps the time has come for America to learn the lesson of the leaves.

CHAPTER THIRTY-ONE

AN AGENDA FOR IMPROVEMENT

To save a person dying of a heart attack, it takes 911, ambulances, EMTs, doctors, nurses, hospitals, researchers, drugs, technicians, supplies, buildings and surgical suites, on and on.

These necessities are expensive to obtain and specialized to the task. They require years to cultivate and organize. Yet they exist, and succeed with astonishing regularity. The point is that society is perfectly capable of marshaling its people, institutions, money, and wit to save lives.

What about when the goal is not saving a life but giving it value? What about when the purpose of care is not cure but comfort? Suddenly these legions of resources for emergency treatment are beside the point. The tools patients need during slow dying are not nearly as complicated or expensive or difficult to organize. For all but the rarest conditions, for example, excellent pain medication already exists. Most patients need little more equipment than a bed. Practitioners of this care must have expertise, but empathy is more essential. Compared with bringing rescue squads to a car crash, extracting injured people, transporting them to a hospital, operating on them, helping them recover, and sending them home with a rehab plan, caring for a person with a slow illness looks easy.

The obstacles clearly are not about techniques or inventions. The real challenges are attitudinal—that people who are dying accept their condition, that loved ones join in that recognition, and especially that society organize itself around the idea that death with dignity is appropriate and attainable.

These ideas are abstract. But there are many concrete steps American society can and should take to make a person's death as meaningful and self-directed as the life he or she lived when healthy.

The agenda below is organized according to which entity could best bring about a particular change. It may be an oversimplification. Whoever bears primary responsibility for an action, better end-of-life care ultimately will require systems as intertwined as the staff of the Greek healing god on the ancient symbol for medicine and the snake coiled around it.

GOVERNMENT

Federal policy regarding end-of-life care has not changed significantly since President Ronald Reagan signed the Medicare hospice benefit into law in 1981. While dying has changed dramatically, government has stood still. The pay that doctors and hospices receive for treating dying people is far too low. The criteria for people to qualify for hospice care are too narrow. Too much of a distinction is drawn between care of the dying and treatment of people with chronic illnesses that are not immediately life-threatening. There ought to be a smoother continuum. Government ought to catch up with the reality of gradual dying that more and more Americans experience every day.

Washington did flirt with action on this front in early 2005, in a move as showy as it was narrow. For the first time in history, Congress convened in a special session to consider a bill that concerned a single person. The resulting law—passed in one day to permit the parents of Terry Schiavo to challenge her feeding-tube removal in federal court—won President George W. Bush's signature with a flourish. Judges in several venues, however, readily dismissed the parents' motions. The U.S. Supreme Court declined six times even to hear the case. That unambiguous outcome signals how unfamiliar Congress is with existing medical law. The court delivered what was virtually a rebuke.

However questionable the merits of Washington's intervention, at least it reflected a recognition that the care of a person who is irrevocably dying is a difficult matter. Resulting public debate served the useful purpose of inspiring many people to establish directives for their end-of-life care.

But that response is little more than a society recoiling in distaste. It falls far shy of the broader initiative as universal an experience as gradual dying deserves. Recall from Chapter 16 the National Institutes of Health's

2004 "state of the science" conference. Experts in care of the dying found conclusively that there is a deficit of knowledge, expertise, research, and attention to this subject. The NIH said that for many areas—communication with patients, the impact on doctors and nurses of providing terminal care, symptom management, alternative therapies, spirituality, the role of families—too little is known and too little is being done.

This conference contrasts with the Schiavo bill in two ways: It did not win headlines, and its work pertained to multitudes. Congress's first course of action, were it to follow the NIH group's credible findings, ought to be funding research. Why, when medical tools have never been better, is there still so much untreated pain? What portion of Alzheimer's patients will face a decision about using a feeding tube, and what is the best way to help patients and families prepare for that predicament? Does America need fewer intensive-care beds? What must change so that doctors can prescribe sufficient pain medication without worrying about criminal prosecution?

Above all, what are the clinical benchmarks for good end-of-life treatment? How can they be established as the national standard of care?

One indicator of how far research lags comes from the Osler study. William Osler, M.D., followed 486 patients as they were dying, documenting their symptoms in detail. In terms of the number of patients, this remains one of the largest studies of its kind. Osler performed his research in 1906.

There have been smaller meaningful studies in recent years, but they resulted in large measure from private funding. The Open Society Institute, backed by billionaire George Soros, and the Robert Wood Johnson Foundation, which has underwritten all manner of medical and policy studies, have essentially been bankrolling Americans' efforts to learn more about how people die—and might die better. From 1995 through 2002, these two organizations lavished more than $300 million into palliative care research, studies of best hospice practices, and more. In 2003 their generosity on these topics came to an end; both organizations purposely change direction every few years. That is why the NIH's call for research funding matters; there is still so much to be learned.

Armed with better data, Congress could begin by revising existing laws to reflect the reality of gradual dying. Regulations directing hospitals to inform every patient about advance directives, for example, have proven ineffective. A brochure buried among other papers does not grab the attention of a person coping with a serious illness. It is going to take more.

The federal government and thirty-eight state legislatures have established patients' bills of rights, protecting the privacy of medical records, mandating access to second opinions, and other assurances. Why not expand these laws to guarantee that dying people receive proper pain management? Why not make the option of hospice a dying person's right?

Maybe that's asking too much, given Congress's inaction in this area for more than twenty-five years. Even without making hospice an explicit right, though, thousands of Americans annually would benefit if Medicare's hospice eligibility grew in several crucial ways. Foremost, doctors should not have to certify that a patient will be dead within six months in order for that person to qualify for end-of-life care at home. This requirement is an ineffective masquerade for medical caution—particularly when home care costs far less than expensive hospital beds and nursing homes.

Besides, voluminous data confirms that doctors are terrible at forecasting when patients will die. Typically they see death as much farther away than it actually is. Partly this tendency is due to denial and partly because some slow illnesses defy prediction. By external measures, on the day before death the typical heart-failure patient still has a 50-50 chance of living for six months. Two weeks from death, 40 percent of people with liver failure from cirrhosis still have health indicators that they might survive six more months. "Death from emphysema is similarly difficult to predict," writes end-of-life-care expert Joanne Lynn, M.D.

No wonder the median U.S. hospice stay has remained steady for almost a decade at about three and a half weeks. Doctors delay prognostication until the dying process is all but complete, thereby robbing patients and their families of months in which they could have benefited from hospice, home care, pain management, and personalized medicine. A person can prepare and resolve and accomplish a great deal in the gap between six months and three and a half weeks.

Moreover, the hospice benefit currently presents too much of an either/or proposition. Federal law requires patients to cease all life-extending care in order to qualify for hospice. Either people undergo chemotherapy, receive dialysis, and accept other life-sustaining treatments, or they have their hospice costs reimbursed. They have to choose. But patients should not have to toss a coin between dialysis and hospice, between palliative care for cancer and earning a few more weeks of life with chemotherapy that slows the disease's advance. A person who wants to die at home should not have to earn that privilege by surrendering all hope of extending life.

The current policy does not exist for the purpose of being inhumane, of course. It is intended as a cost control, a means of concentrating the demands that hospice care generates for nurses and aides in the last portion of life. Moreover, in the early years of federally supported hospice in the United States, there were issues of potential financial fraud.

It is therefore a plausible argument that the Medicare system cannot afford the expense of catering to people who are dying. It is already under financial strain. Expanding eligibility and reimbursing doctors for helping patients to plan their care will cost money.

But numerous studies have found that hospice actually saves money, by reducing people's use of hospital beds, labs, technicians, and intensive-care units. More than 90 percent of people who establish advance directives do so to set limits on their treatment, thus curbing use of medical resources.

Can America afford better end-of-life care? One answer lies in Great Britain. Granted, that nation has a different health system—one that is government-run as opposed to the market forces of insurers and providers in the United States. Still, Britain's first hospice opened years before any in the country. If England's economy can withstand the expense of caring well for people near the end of their lives, so can America's.

What is fitting for seniors through Medicare is also appropriate for people who are not in that program. Private health insurers need incentives to provide a better hospice benefit. Too many cover only a brief period or a severely limited dollar amount. Whether through the carrot of tax breaks or the stick of a mandate, Congress must inspire the health-insurance industry to adopt policies that reflect how dying has changed.

Action on this front may be inevitable. Hospice must thrive because the United States cannot afford the alternative. With a rapidly growing elderly population, with an ever larger share of lives ending gradually, with such a staggering portion of health-care dollars spent on the last months and weeks of life, and with 83 percent of the people who die today covered by Medicare, this equation is fiscally insupportable.

Already the family's role in caregiving is leading to bankruptcies. Already Medicare is struggling with deficits, paying only a fraction of its beneficiaries' medical costs. Already those unpaid costs are shifted onto the medical bills of people who have health insurance, resulting in premium increases at double the rate of inflation annually.

This country simply must improve end-of-life care, or face stratospheric federal deficits. Inaction is a luxury America cannot afford.

WHILE AWAITING FEDERAL REMEDIES, state governments can take a more aggressive role on their own.

California, for example, enacted a law requiring doctors to receive training in pain management. The mandate has thus far proved both successful for patients and less onerous than physicians had feared.

Doctors renew their licenses every two years. What California did was require doctors to complete a brief course in managing patients' pain as a condition of renewal. To describe physicians' initial opinion of this idea as opposed would be an understatement. To characterize most doctors' attitudes before the training as reluctant would be comical. But when doctors were asked their views after the program, nearly all declared it time well spent. They discovered how little they knew about pain control and how much better they could do the job. A similar proposal for nurses is gaining political momentum. Every state can benefit from California's example. There is no excuse for a doctor to be ignorant in the treatment of pain.

Another way states can foster better end-of-life care comes from Oregon. In each state there is an oversight board that handles patient complaints against physicians, meting out discipline if warranted. For a doctor to be sanctioned, the board must find that he or she failed to meet the established standard of care. When it comes to pain management, that bar is too low. Any competent lawyer can defend a doctor with the argument that the standard of care for pain management is to undertreat it. Thus, doctors who ignore patients' suffering receive no sanctions.

Yet there are glimmers of change. In 1999 Oregon's board of physician regulation encountered the case of pulmonary specialist Paul Bilder, M.D., of Roseburg. His treatment of dying patients' pain drew a disciplinary inquiry. The state's charges allege this history of conduct:

- Treating an elderly man with prostate and lung cancer, Bilder gave him Tylenol and later Darvocet. When a hospice nurse complained, Bilder "ordered substantially inadequate amounts of pain medication." The patient died the next day.

- The family of an eighty-four-year-old man with lung cancer and urinary incontinence asked that he receive a catheter. A nurse granted that request, but Bilder ordered that it be removed and the patient use diapers. The nurse requested oral morphine; Bilder approved a fraction of the request. The patient died that night.

- A thirty-five-year-old woman with respiratory disease and other conditions came to the hospital and was placed on a ventilator, with sedatives and pain medication. Bilder discontinued the sedative and pain drugs. The patient removed the breathing tube herself, and Bilder ordered a paralytic drug so the woman could not do it again, but not a sedative for anxiety over shortness of breath.

- A sixty-three-year-old woman with lung disease came to Bilder's hospital with respiratory failure. She was put on a ventilator. Bilder refused a request for more pain medication, instead ordering that the patient be paralyzed "without any sedatives or pain medication."

- An eighty-two-year-old man with congestive heart failure arrived at Bilder's hospital with difficulty breathing. Bilder declined to administer pain medication despite repeated requests. Eventually another doctor treated the patient, who stabilized and went home several days later.

- A thirty-three-year-old man with pneumonia came to the hospital. Bilder's attempts to place the breathing tube through the patient's nose caused bleeding, but he did not use anti-anxiety drugs or pain medication. The patient, who became "combative" from oxygen hunger, was physically restrained.

The allegations were never prosecuted; Bilder settled the case first. He kept his medical license, but regulators required him to enroll in a peer-evaluation program, complete a course in patient-physician communication, and receive psychiatric care.

It was the first and only known case of a physician being disciplined because of ill treatment of patients' pain. Some end-of-life-care advocates made much of that precedent, but it is fair to ask if the sanction worked. In 2003 the board disciplined Bilder again.

This time, the state charged, Bilder treated a patient with advanced cancer by giving him Tylenol #3. When the patient complained of "severe pain whenever he moved," Bilder had an angry confrontation with a hospice nurse. After increasing the patient's pain medication to include Oxycodone, he noted in the patient's chart that further treatment "would just prolong things."

Another patient, who had breast cancer, was hospitalized for delirium and pain for months. After the pain increased, Bilder gave her a patch that would not take effect for eight to twelve hours, as well as some liquid morphine. When the patient groaned, Bilder "informed the nurse that groaning does not necessarily mean the patient is in pain." The patient died five days later.

These charges, too, are only allegations; Bilder again settled the case before prosecution. Regulators gave him a public reprimand, placed him on probation for ten years, required monitoring his care of terminally ill patients, and ordered him to continue receiving psychiatric care. Again Bilder kept his medical license. He still has it today.

If Oregon's sanction was too light, at least it represented progress. The notion of holding doctors accountable for patients' pain could spread. The fifty states' medical boards belong to a national association, primarily to keep a doctor disciplined in one state from simply moving to another one and practicing there. Following the Bilder case, several state medical boards began establishing pain-management rules, with a focus on terminal patients. The association has also begun workshops to help state boards oversee pain-management issues consistently. These initiatives could become national in reach without requiring any new laws, if state medical boards act within their powers to declare a standard of care and then hold doctors to it.

There's another way regulators can make a difference without waiting for new laws. Study upon study has found that doctors routinely ignore patients' advance directives. However, physicians bear no accountability for that misdeed. State medical boards could embark on a public education campaign to teach health consumers that advance directives have legal weight. Then, if people file a complaint against a doctor for ignoring their wishes or those of a loved one, the boards could discipline the doctor. Such action would not necessarily help that person, but it would increase the likelihood that future patients receive the care they want.

America's physicians need to see only a handful of their peers disciplined for undertreating pain or ignoring advance directives before their behavior would begin to change.

To be fair, physicians make two cogent arguments against advance directives. First, doctors say the instructions are often vague, don't apply to many situations, or even contain contradictory demands. Since dying is a public health issue, though, it is incumbent upon state health departments to work with doctors to establish reliable, standard language for advance directives that they can provide to patients, lawyers, and others who advocate for people with a terminal illness.

Second, medical teams complain that they have no way of knowing whether a person has an advance directive in place. EMTs arrive at a car accident to find a person whose heart has stopped. Their training is to start that heart again and sort out later whether a ventilator or CPR was welcome.

There is no reason that the good intentions of rescue personnel should be pitted against the legitimate desires of patients. A little creativity could solve the problem. For example, in several states there is a box on the back of the driver's license that a person can check to show that he is willing to be an organ donor. How difficult would it be to add another box, indicating whether the person has an advance directive? A small space naming the doctor, lawyer, or friend possessing that document would help EMTs provide care the patient actually wants.

The next suggestion comes with an admitted caution. It pertains to how health consumers can use courts to enhance the medical world's sensitivity to suffering. Perhaps those who receive lousy care should sue.

The immediate danger of this suggestion lies in encouraging legal action in a society that already is too litigious. Doctors today practice a kind of defensive medicine, aiming to protect themselves and their careers while treating patients. The simplest example is the change in what a hospital medical chart contains. Traditionally this clipboard has reflected a patient's clinical situation, physicians' orders, and nurses' observations. Now the chart serves the additional purpose of establishing documentation for any potential future lawsuit. This is one small illustration of how the culture in which doctors and nurses do their jobs is shifting, not away from patient care necessarily but toward a place burdened with defensiveness and worry nonetheless. This reality has driven physicians out of the profession, has made health care more costly because of needless defensive medicine, and has increased doctors' malpractice insurance expenses. The fraction of malpractice suits that are frivolous has even fostered a backlash against appropriate use of the courts by wronged health consumers. Thus, any proposal that people should sue comes advisedly.

Still, there are examples of how courts can send a powerful message.

One came in 1991, in North Carolina. An elderly man named Henry James was terminally ill with prostate cancer. He entered a nursing home with a prescription for opioid pain drugs—morphine, perhaps, or oxycodone. The supervising nurse refused to administer Henry's prescription, however, because in her professional opinion it would lead to his addiction. She gave him a mild tranquilizer instead, which did not relieve his pain. After Henry died, his family sued the nurse and the nursing home. The jury awarded $7.5 million in compensatory damages and $7.5 million in punitive damages.

In California eighty-five-year-old William Bergman was admitted to Eden Medical Center in Castro Valley in 1998 in the care of Wing Chin, M.D. William entered the hospital because of stress fractures in his back, but doctors discovered that he had lung cancer.

He was also in pain. For his six days in the hospital, on a scale of 1 to 10 (with 10 being worst), William consistently reported a level of discomfort of 7 or higher. When he was discharged from the hospital, he reported being at 10. William died at home three days later.

His three children sued, alleging that Chin had committed elder abuse by not giving their father sufficient pain medication. Uniquely, California law permits such suits. The standard of proof is appreciably higher than a regular malpractice suit, though; plaintiffs must prove not merely that the doctor was "negligent" but that he was "reckless."

An Alameda County superior court jury found that Chin was indeed reckless, awarding the family $1.5 million. The final amount will likely be less after appeals, because California limits the size of awards in these suits. Money is not the point, anyway; accountability is.

Both generous verdicts indicate how intensely juries scowl upon medical professionals and institutions that treat patients' pain with insufficient regard. The California lawsuit has special merit because the Bergman family also filed a complaint with the state board that regulates doctors, which took no action against Chin. Suing was the only remedy left to the family of a man who had suffered needlessly.

It is worth repeating that America does not need a wave of lawsuits to clog overburdened courts and increase health-care costs. Also, doctors who provide appropriate pain control deserve a clear signal from their government that keeping a dying person comfortable will not land them in jail. Still, when research finds people enduring so much preventable pain, litigation may accelerate the pace of systemic change.

Behind the various policy ideas—regulation, lawsuits, boxes on licenses—lurks a larger principle: Although death is a consummately private act, it occurs in a context of practices, finances, and laws that unquestionably make it a public health issue. The number of people suffering to death each year, the impact gradual dying has on families, the fiscal consequences when one-third of Medicare spending goes to the last year of people's lives—these issues manifest across society. So, whether the initiative comes from a state health department, a department of motor vehicles, a physician oversight board, Congress, or the White House, government possesses many tools to improve people's lives at a crucial time.

One further contribution by government is essential: leadership. All policy ideas aside, sometimes the nation needs political leaders to exercise the bully pulpit that their position provides. Imagine, for example, if President Bush, upon signing the Schiavo bill in 2005, had immediately also signed his own advance directive—right there, in front of the cameras. The impact would have been profound, sparking an enlightened debate. Imagine if the surgeon general next conducted a national dialogue on end-of-life care, modeled on President Clinton's race initiative in the 1990s. Such initiatives would make something constructive out of the demagoguery over Terry Schiavo. Instead of words and poses, action.

The need for leadership on end-of-life care is long overdue. True, a few members of Congress are loyal allies of hospice. But hearings like those that shaped the 1970s debate over access to dialysis, when that treatment was new, simply have not occurred. The voice with national reach that can articulate end-of-life issues in the political realm has thus far been silent.

Perhaps what is needed is experience. Maybe the leadership will arise once enough members of Congress have watched their own loved ones suffer their way to the grave.

THE MEDICAL COMMUNITY

Medical training in death and dying is plainly inadequate. Only a handful of medical schools require detailed study of pain control. Most limit the subject to one textbook chapter, though pain relief is often the most urgent issue patients have—and is a primary need of people who are dying.

Medical schools deemphasize care for people who are terminally ill, if they mention it at all. In some schools death, though it affects every patient, receives less attention than infectious diseases that do not even occur on this continent. Medical schools need new priorities. This is not to say that changing the curriculum will be easy, only that it is necessary.

Meanwhile, there is an acute need for training practicing physicians in palliative and hospice care. Postresidency fellowships in pain management and terminal care are overdue as well. Those programs that do exist reach too few doctors. The American Board of Medical Specialties needs to make palliative care a recognized, reimbursable specialty—with all the professional standing of orthopedics, pediatrics, or gynecology.

Through such advances, physicians who concentrate in end-of-life medicine would establish a standard of care for their generalist peers. Such enhancements would also heighten the status of doctors who care for people who are dying, leading to increased research funding—and in the long-term an increased likelihood that patients receive competent attention.

As the emphasis shifts, there will be greater incentives for researchers to write better medical textbooks and for publishers to offer them. When medical students of the future encounter material unknown to today's students, a cycle of improvement will begin.

The improvement has already begun in a few places. Missoula, Montana, has an exemplary hospice. Pittsburgh, Pennsylvania, has a fast-growing clinical and research program in end-of-life care. Certain counties in Florida do an exceptional job for people who are dying slowly.

Some hospitals, too, have developed programs that make a difference.

- The Veterans Affairs Medical Center in Dayton, Ohio, set out to increase advance-care planning for patients with lung cancer, congestive heart failure, or chronic obstructive pulmonary disease. They produced an informational video, distributed a patient-education booklet, opened an advance-planning clinic, and started a bereavement support group. Twelve weeks later advance-care planning had leapt from 15 percent of patients to nearly 90 percent.

- The M. D. Anderson Cancer Center in Houston gave doctors a "breaking bad news" workshop. Then patients took a survey of their satisfaction with those conversations, helping the doctors improve.

- The University of Utah Hospital in Salt Lake City concentrated on grief. They made it hospital policy to send a "thinking of you" card to families of patients who had died, calling to say a packet of helpful resources was on its way and sending the information about ways people grieve and a directory of local bereavement services.

There are comparable examples of effective physician education in end-of-life care. After only modest exposure to caring for the dying, medical students, residents, and seasoned doctors alike confirmed personal and professional gains. Many of these men and women reawakened to the empathy that led them to choose a medical career.

For the most part, though, these programs are small and brief. Similarly, the islands of excellence in end-of-life care exist primarily because of local factors. There is some expert, some charismatic leader, or some local demographic idiosyncrasy that explains the high quality of care. That's wonderful for the people who happen to live there. But the medical community needs comparably high standards that are systemic, turning the practices of the best places into procedures and attitudes across the country.

The Joint Commission on Accreditation of Healthcare Organizations is one leadership body that is trying. JCAHO is the national accrediting organization for hospitals, nursing homes, and rehabilitation centers. When JCAHO inspects an institution, it means months of preparation, an anxious week during the review, and crossed fingers until JCAHO announces its results. If JCAHO finds a deficient area of care, it can order a hospital to change practices that range from where supplies are kept to how hiring is done. A hospital must comply promptly, or its accreditation is at risk.

In 2000, JCAHO began devoting greater attention to pain relief, in palliative care and throughout the health system. "Patients have the right to pain management," JCAHO has declared. It established a requirement for accreditation that a hospital "respects and supports" that right.

To that end, JCAHO dubbed pain "the fifth vital sign." For decades medicine has monitored the four key indicators of a patient's condition: heart rate, breathing rate, temperature, and blood pressure. JCAHO sought to give patients' pain as high a status as the beating of their hearts.

That view may be appropriate for people in their lives' last chapter, because they have so many nonmedical needs. You cannot tackle emotional issues until you conquer the physical ones. You can't arrange your finances if you can't think clearly. You can't resolve relationships while distracted by physical suffering. You can't dance until your feet stop hurting.

Symbolically, therefore, JCAHO's move was first-rate. Substantively, there's room for improvement. The heat has gone out of the initiative, and the people who developed the pain-control standards are no longer with the organization. Meanwhile, in 2004 problems with pain management were the fifth-leading issue uncovered in JCAHO's reviews of hospitals.

There's a reason that concentrating on hospitals makes sense: At this point not enough of the U.S. population dies to warrant establishing universal access to hospice care. About 850,000 Americans a year could benefit from hospice services, which does not justify creating an entirely new clinical infrastructure. An intermediate move—which costs less and takes an evolutionary step toward dignified dying—is to provide palliative care within existing facilities. Today 80 percent of U.S. hospitals remain without a palliative-care service.

They may not know how many incentives they have to act. Researchers at St. John's Regional Medical Center in Joplin, Missouri, measured the financial difference that palliative care could make. Tracking 197 patients between October 2000 and April 2002, they found a savings of $315,915. How did it happen? Patients received treatments at the appropriate place, which meant shorter ICU stays. Also, because good palliative care includes preparing for possible crises, patients' care was better managed. That made it less expensive.

Additionally, doctors, nurses, and social workers were better supported in their work. Families were involved in care management. And all the while, patients received better care.

"Medicine evolved throughout the centuries by concentrating narrowly and deeply on one dimension of personhood—the body," write doctors at the Mayo Clinic in Rochester, Minnesota.

"The implication is that by knowing the body and disease on a detailed molecular level, physicians know about suffering. . . . Well-meaning physicians find that spending the time necessary to address 'whole person needs' creates economic and professional risk. Thus physicians continue to focus on the physical aspect. When their patients suffer, physicians seek a physical solution. When more than pain medication is needed, however, physicians have had little else to offer.

"When attempting to know what makes people suffer and understanding the means to alleviate that suffering, medicine frequently misses the point."

The medical community needs to get the point, and right away, for reasons that cut to the profession's *moral* foundation. Granted, it is dangerous to assert moral absolutes with a topic as complex as gradual dying. For some people, anything other than prolonging life by all possible means is immoral. For others, lavishing limited health-care resources on people whose time is dwindling is immoral. Yet both camps may agree—and be joined by people of more moderate views—on four moral imperatives that the health system simply must answer:

Expertise. Each patient experiences his dying only once. Families rarely see the end of more than two or three lives. But doctors witness death all the time. That disparity in expertise creates an implicit responsibility. It is the doctor's job to accept when dying has begun. It is the expert's task to tell patients and families the truth. It is the physician's role to anticipate problems and help people plan in advance in case these situations arise.

This responsibility may create awkwardness, if not deep discomfort. For that, physicians deserve our sympathy as well as systems to support them in times of difficulty. They do not, however, deserve absolution from the responsibilities of a role they have chosen for themselves.

Informed consent. It is a rightly accepted tenet in medicine that respect for the personal autonomy of patients requires that they freely choose whether or not to receive care. Aside from emergencies, people cannot undergo surgery without signing a form that says they acknowledge the risks and give their consent. Yet millions of patients today embark on care for terminal illness—organ failure, cancer, Alzheimer's—far from fully informed about what may happen and what their options are.

What goes for surgery must also go for ventilators and feeding tubes. If the medical community genuinely believes in informed consent, it must radically change its communication with people who are dying.

Genuine consent means informing patients about alternatives, too. The question is not "Do you want the tube to help your breathing?" Informed patients would know their odds of needing a ventilator, prospects for recovery once that point arrives, other paths they might take, and what would minimize the distress of choosing not to be put on a ventilator.

In general, a higher priority must be placed not only on telling the truth but also on telling it earlier. Even when the topic is death, the American public can handle it. Indeed, given the empowered consumers people have become, they will welcome it.

Pain. There is simply no excuse today for people to live their final weeks and hours in pain. None. The technology is there, the drugs exist, the cost is not exorbitant. The public needs to learn how minimal the potential is for terminal patients to become addicted to pain medicines. Law-enforcement leaders bear responsibility for working with physicians to ensure that legitimate crime fighting does not impede legitimate patient care. The alleviation of suffering ought to be medicine's foremost purpose.

Alternatives. Today's insufficient end-of-life care does not occur in a political vacuum. Health consumers are increasingly aware of proposals for physician-assisted suicide and euthanasia. They know that these notions have taken hold in other countries, that Oregon has approved assisted suicide, that other states have contemplated this dramatic step. The medical community has spoken vehemently against these proposals. The American Medical Association and advocates for people who are disabled have stood shoulder to shoulder against assisted suicide. They argue that hastening a patient's dying perverts the role of the physician, from healer to instrument of death. They say people who ask a doctor to end their life nearly always drop that request once they receive proper care.

These organizations' stances, while sustained and sincere, will not prevail forever. The longer the health system takes to improve care of the dying, the weaker its arguments against alternatives become. Americans will not continue to suffer, nor watch loved ones suffer, while doctors and hospitals and medical schools dither. If the public becomes convinced that ending a patient's life is the only way to end his or her agony, they will open the door to extreme measures. The political clock is ticking.

There are many other moral dimensions pertaining to end-of-life care, but it is more appealing to consider instead what might happen if doctors, nurses, policy makers, and the administrators of health institutions accept just these four challenges. The resulting human potential is nigh unlimited.

One encouraging story of that potential comes from Canada, where a plan to propagate palliative care saw failure, then success, then a stunning appearance of so many meaningful aftereffects that researchers later described the result as "serendipitous ripples."

The Institute of Palliative Care in Ottawa wanted to teach community doctors how to deliver competent care to people who are dying. They devised a comprehensive curriculum, won funding from the Ontario Ministry of Health and Long-Term Care, and established a stellar two-week educational program.

It bombed. Over a three-year span only twenty-two doctors took part.

While saying they had learned a great deal, the doctors reported frustration with implementing those lessons in their communities. They felt isolated, too, disconnected from local colleagues who had not bought into the palliative and home-care concepts.

To their credit, the institute's educators changed direction. They held focus groups with doctors. They learned that asking a physician to take two weeks away from his practice was simply too much. Then they rebuilt the program. Now each community—doctors, nurses, home-care organizations, long-term care groups, and volunteer organizers—would develop its own list of educational needs. The institute would work with each community to develop thirty-hour educational programs that contained common core material but also elements responding to the local needs. The institute's goal was to engage forty to sixty physicians over two years, but responsibility for recruiting them was left to local leaders.

The goals were not ambitious enough. In all, 114 doctors, plus 187 nurses and other health workers, took part. The sessions involved solving problems in small, interdisciplinary groups—just as people do with real patients. Leading local doctors designed additional ten-hour intensives to fill gaps in their knowledge and established links with the institute's experts for whenever a consultation might be needed.

That would have been success enough. Instead, things were just becoming interesting.

First, at the systemic level, the local participants decided on their own initiative to keep meeting, brainstorming to improve palliative care in their communities. Local groups also identified the need for better spiritual care for patients. Generalist doctors voiced problems they had communicating with cancer specialists, which led to creation of a "nurse navigator" to serve as intermediary and ombudsman.

Second, at the local level, doctors who had taken the institute's course informed their colleagues, then watched their palliative care referrals more than triple in three years. Phone contacts between local doctors and the institute more than doubled. Regional palliative care experts said they were able to stop visits at some local hospitals because their advice was no longer needed. Long-term care workers reported greater consistency in doctors' orders for pain management. In one community a theater group became involved, producing a show about a family in distress over a loved one's terminal illness—which was videotaped for use as another educational tool.

Third, at the individual level, people who took the course said it affected them personally. One physician wrote to the faculty "express-ing how the knowledge she had gained from the program allowed her to care for a patient with terminal thyroid cancer and to fulfill the patient's wish to die peacefully at home surrounded by her family." Another said the program had helped her cope with a terminal illness in her own family.

So many "serendipitous ripples." These energized health practition-ers, once they were properly educated in palliative care, went well beyond anyone's hopes or expectations. The ultimate winners, of course, were patients, who received better care at a critical time in their lives.

That was Ottawa. Yet American health institutions also possess the resources, intellect, and medical capacity to make this kind of success a commonplace achievement. Imagine a day when helping a dying person breathe well, or vanquishing her pain, or helping her decide what kind of care she wants should her condition deteriorate, becomes as ordinary as setting a broken arm, stitching a cut, giving a child a vaccine.

To shorten the distance between that prospect and the state of affairs today, it is not a matter of skill. It is a matter of will.

THE MERITS OF PROPER end-of-life care do not begin and end with that fraction of patients whose life has entered the last chapter. Principles of palliative thinking can be applied beneficially to every branch of medicine.

Why should only doctors and nurses make observations on a patient's medical chart? Why can't the patient and his family? Why should a pa-tient who can walk be required to leave the hospital by wheelchair? What can be done to make patients less passive in medical situations and more active participants in their care? Why do patients who are not contagious nonetheless eat in the solitude of their rooms rather than in more social settings like cafeterias? Why must hospital patients continue to wear bed-clothes that minimize dignity and individuality?

For all its stunning advances in technology, knowledge, and proce-dures, health care in general would be handsomely enriched by greater emphasis on the patient as a person rather than as a manifestation of ill-ness; by renewed attention to people's comfort as an essential dimension of their condition; by enhanced understanding of a person's life outside of the illness and the clinical setting; by acceptance of the limits of medical science; by humility in the face of what awaits us all; by a sharpened sense of collaboration among medical professionals, patients, and fami-

lies; and by deeper respect for the spiritual dimensions of life and its ultimate mysteries.

Humanizing the scientific does not require sacrificing any tools or tests
or techniques. But greater empathy and compassion enriches the power of
those tools and makes larger the hearts of the people who use them.

THE AMERICAN PUBLIC

When the new interstate highways brought soaring auto fatalities in the
1960s, President Johnson called for creation of what later became EMTs.
A massive mobilization began. That so many Americans now survive
causes of sudden death proves that this nation's culture is capable of reacting to a complex medical challenge in a constructive and effective way.

The time for another sweeping change has come. The need grows
more pressing with every new case of Alzheimer's disease, every kidney
failure, every new HIV infection, every cancer diagnosis. The challenges
for Americans lie in looking beyond the isolating sorrow of deaths they
have seen, realizing that their experience is not unique, and then recognizing how the road to that place could have been so much smoother. The
incredible power of emotions surrounding loss, once they are turned toward positive change, will be a juggernaut.

TO ACCOMPLISH THE INITIAL step of heightening public attention, numerous organizations equipped for the job are standing by. But their sepa-
rate energies, which sometimes compete, first must be joined. The
American Heart Association, American Lung Association, American
Cancer Society, and their many brethren organizations all have done great
deeds to raise awareness of the needs of people with those illnesses. However, they also vie against one another for research dollars and visibility.
Since nearly all of them have policies supporting improved end-of-life
care, their combined effort would be a formidable political force.

Who might link these groups? The American Medical Association
could go beyond its supportive policy statements and invest genuine
physician leadership. The American Association of Retired Persons,
which boasts millions of members and is rarely shy about flexing its political muscle, might provide a political hub around which the disease-
advocacy groups could effectively turn.

Service organizations could contribute, too. Local Red Cross chapters, YMCAs, and other groups routinely offer courses such as water safety and CPR. These programs, while worthy, need to evolve to reflect today's medical reality. Instead of a half-day CPR class, what if one of these organizations instead offered a half-day introduction to hospice? As an alternative to junior lifesaving, what about senior caretaking?

Professionals have a part to play as well. The American Bar Association could do more to encourage its lawyer-members to include, in their work on wills, helping clients write advance directives. The life-insurance industry could remind its customers that financial preparation is a close cousin to medical preparation. Malpractice insurers could reward doctors who develop expertise in reducing patient suffering and helping families, because those steps reduce the likelihood of a subsequent lawsuit. In fact, the leading malpractice insurer in Colorado does just that, offering discounts to doctors who take courses in pain management.

Business organizations could also participate. The Leapfrog Group, for example, is a business initiative to improve the caliber of U.S. health care. So far the group, which consists of many of the nation's largest employers, has drawn worthwhile attention to reducing medical errors in hospitals. But Leapfrog and its peers have yet to weigh in on how to improve care for people beginning their final journey. These groups—in intellect, energy, and clout—have much to contribute.

THE GREATEST GAINS will occur once medical consumers awaken to how dying has changed, and begin to advocate on their own behalf. It could be an issue that appeals to men, because they die on average about five years younger than women and they could take greater responsibility for themselves. Conversely, at Americans for Better Care of the Dying in Washington, D.C., end-of-life care is a feminist issue. Too often women provide final caretaking, see their spouse die, then come home from the funeral to discover that the money they had planned to live on for the rest of their days has all been spent. "This caretaking role, which is predominantly done by women, is one of the fastest growing causes of elderly impoverishment," said Dr. Joanne Lynn.

The issue is larger than gender, though. Baby boomers, 47 million strong, are beginning to experience the death of their parents. They are therefore learning firsthand how dying has changed. Given the bold personality of this giant demographic group—they have transformed public attitudes toward large institutions, sexuality, organized religion, traditional family structures, and more—they are bound to assert themselves on their ill parents' behalf. With the high value baby boomers place on autonomy, they are virtually certain to learn from their parents' suffering and to demand more dignified dying for themselves.

They can start by ignoring arguments that health care is too complex to change. Recall in the early 1990s, when managed-care companies were permitting only twenty-four-hour hospital stays for new mothers—what some called "drive-by deliveries." During the debate it did not matter how much longer hospital stays would cost. It did not even matter that some studies found better health outcomes for mothers and babies if they went home sooner. Baby boomers cried out for forty-eight-hour hospital stays, government mandated it, and that became the standard of care.

There are countless other examples of the health-care system acceding to consumer demands—health insurance plans adding erectile-dysfunction drugs to their formulary, birth-control pills also being added, certain pain drugs being removed after a few notorious cases of abuse.

Several million noisy health consumers would help improve end-of-life care in much the same way. America has accomplished this before, developing emergency medicine when death was sudden. It can happen again. Ideal end-of-life care need not be a dream.

WHEN THE AMERICAN CULTURE around dying shifts, it will improve medicine, cost less, and help families. But the largest impact will be on patients themselves.

"Dying is an inherently lonely state, because it is irreversible, relentless, incomparable in its finality, and because social support typically comes from persons, albeit empathetic, not experiencing dying." So write doctors on the New York Medical Society's Committee on Bioethical Issues.

"Patients' concerns about burdening loved ones are potent values in settings of poor prognosis," add UCLA researchers who interviewed elderly Californians. "Concerns about family burden are a principal reason that patients reject life-sustaining treatments."

Yes, people literally would rather die than inconvenience their family. Another survey found that one of the primary reasons patients ask for physician-assisted suicide is the fear of being a burden on family members.

This attitude is more profound than simple pride. When very sick people refuse support, it works both as a defense against admitting that they are dying and as an effort to protect those they love. Patients do not want to be a burden in part because it will tax their family and in part because to do so would signify that they have begun an irreversible process.

Here's the opposite possibility: The more American society awakens to the value of giving people a better final journey, and the more that families and physicians alike experience the gratification of succeeding in that effort, the more comfortable patients will become in asking for and accepting support. People who are dying can learn that allowing someone to help does not inflict a burden. Rather, it bestows a privilege, an ultimate intimacy, a series of images and experiences that endure in the caregiver's life forever. Patients who surrender to this reality even find that their medical care improves.

That's not just sentiment. The UCLA researchers confirm it. "Acts of caring—relieving burdens and strengthening relationships with loved ones—are critical to patients' perceptions of quality end-of-life care," they write. The researchers therefore suggest that "in situations where patients' prognosis for recovery is poor, physicians would recognize the importance that caretaking behaviors play within families, and would actively support family members' desire to care for their dying loved one."

For Reverend Donald Moore, a theology professor in New York City, a patient who lets others help does more than improve his or her own experience. "I see death not only as an opportunity to reflect on the meaning of your own existence, but to offer your life as a gift to others."

There are three ways of putting that idea into action. The first is for patients to insist on dignified care, to demand pain control, to set a standard for their care that is higher than the status quo, to instruct everyone within earshot about the value of living well for as long as possible. Such consumer demands would drive changes in medical conduct faster than any other force.

The second is for people to take greater responsibility for their well-being. That means creating a health-care proxy so someone can speak on their behalf. This is not a matter of inviting death; it is simple self-protection. Poor Terry Schiavo spent fifteen years on a feeding tube while her husband and parents debated its removal. One signed piece of paper would have prevented the whole ordeal. Anyone who wants to avoid a similar fate ought to take an hour preparing such a paper.

The third step is for people to reflect on their power to shape the experience of those around them. Do they want their loved ones to feel pushed away, held at arm's length? Or when their time on earth has ended, do they want to leave their friends and families with a sense of accomplishment, of gratification, of having made a difference?

REFORMING END-OF-LIFE CARE is bound to be controversial. Proposals for change will meet resistance. There will be winners and losers. The health industry is not nimble, and billions of dollars are invested in the tools and facilities that deliver life-prolonging care today. For example, there are 60,826 intensive care beds in America's hospitals. Each one requires expensive equipment; technicians to operate and maintain the machinery; doctors, nurses, and their managers. If more Americans embrace hospice, dying at home with their medical care limited to pain control, the financial fallout could be massive. Hospital administrators will not twiddle their thumbs while ventilators stand idle.

Yet the need for a less costly approach grows more urgent with each day that baby boomers age. More important than money, however, is the human cost. Every day thousands of people across the country are experiencing the wrong kind of final chapter—needlessly painful, fruitlessly prolonged, dehumanizing and undignified. Millions of Americans are learning that the agonies of dying in this manner are preventable, and that helping a person to end life in peace is much harder than it needs to be.

CHAPTER THIRTY-TWO

FOUR FINAL LESSONS

Changes in end-of-life care are sure to come, as thousands of Americans witness dying's new form and are hurt by its consequences. A nation founded on liberty and self-determination will not suffer without taking action.

But as government policy, medical education, and the American public work on improvements, they will encounter four important—perhaps life-changing—lessons about the art of dying that transcend this moment in history, speaking to something more enduring and elemental. For each of the four, in my case, the research for this book provided clear instruction.

FIRST THERE IS THE LESSON from Bruce Fonda, Ph.D., professor of gross anatomy at the University of Vermont's College of Medicine for more than twenty years. I went to him hoping to learn the basics of dissection class; instead, I received an education about the true nature of our mortality.

I interviewed Bruce one bright September day. His office had a pelvis on the shelf; a skeleton named Killer hung behind my chair. The name is not about death, Fonda said, but about the incredibly hard exam in which students must name all of his bones and their related nerves and arteries.

He instructed me for hours about medical memorization, what kind of person donates his body, how students process the experience of disassembling a corpse. Bruce was guarded, making sure I understood the respect with which cadavers are treated. Once I passed his scrutiny he showed me the refrigerator room, where plastic-wrapped bodies lay on rows of racks. Bruce took me to the dissection lab, afternoon sun pouring through its western windows. On a side table, a brain, spinal cord, and all the major nerves lay bathed in clear solution in a long plastic container. "That's about eighty hours' work," he said.

Soon Bruce handed me a heart. Its exterior had been sliced so he could pinkie it open and show me the network of arteries and veins within. It is no small thing to hold a human heart in your hand. Next he gave me a heart enlarged by disease, and I could see for myself the tidy blue thread where a valve replacement had occurred in some long-past time. I opened the ventricle and poked my finger through the plastic valve a surgeon had installed, to prolong the life of this heart's former person. The valve opened and closed like the hinged cover atop a bulldozer's exhaust pipe.

Eventually I worked up the nerve to ask Bruce if he had any aortas. From a cabinet, he produced a tub not unlike a cafeteria-size peanut butter container. He lifted the top and handed me a pink tube, perhaps sixteen inches long, thinner in sidewall than a garden hose but nearly as large in diameter.

"This one's a beauty," he said. "You could drop a quarter down that hole."

I imagined a river of blood coursing through that pink tube. The aorta was soft but, I learned by tugging on it, not delicate. I asked if he had one with an abdominal aneurysm.

"A triple-A? I think so."

A moment later it lay in my hand. The tube had a thing growing on the side of it two-thirds of the way down, a knob like the fat burls that grow on old oak trees. It was hard and furled like brain coral.

"It's a fairly good specimen," Bruce said. "This blood vessel's owner was in serious danger."

I was quiet a minute. I was wondering about my father as I stood there holding the cause of his dying. Would he be proud of me now?

"I know what you're thinking," Bruce said.

"Do you?"

"I bet you're thinking that the human body is an incredibly intricate and mysterious machine."

Yes, but that's not all. I was thinking, too, about how this stranger's aorta somehow was linking me to my father in a new and odd way, by revealing the instrument of his death.

Above all, I was contemplating how we are at all times bearing our mortality around with us inside, waiting. We don't know which body part's failure will be the one to finish us, but it is in there right now nonetheless.

"Something like that," I replied. And I handed back to Bruce what my father had never known.

LESSON TWO IS ABOUT GEOFF, managing editor at a newspaper where I once worked and for three years my direct boss. Geoff is an excellent story editor, and generally I was one of his better reporters. Yet he and I got along about as well as two porcupines in a duffel bag. Clashing egos, bad chemistry, whatever you might call it—we bickered, we interrupted, we disparaged each other's ideas. Sometimes we would blow up in fits of temper we never experienced with anyone else.

Then Geoff's wife was diagnosed with breast cancer. Doctors found it had spread to her lymph system, too. The odds in those cases are terrible. She and Geoff have three kids.

Suddenly I could no more argue with Geoff than I could slap a child. The ache of possible death was all around him, in his face and his posture and the surrounding air. It softened him. It softened me, too. In the place that had been occupied by conflict, a friendship flowed in. His wife underwent chemotherapy and radiation, and now lives in that scary limbo of waiting for a clean bill of health at five years. Meanwhile, the friendship has remained.

Lesson two, then, is that death teaches us compassion.

This lesson goes far beyond my one experience. After all, every person is going to die. And every person is going to witness the death of people they love. Thus, each person contains the means of calling forth our compassion, if only we can see the mortality that abides within him or her.

Here is a way to test this notion: Think of a person with whom you have conflict. Now give that person, or someone dear to him, an imaginary terminal illness. Does your attitude toward him soften? Is he more vulnerable? Are your feelings humbler, and more calm?

Follow this idea to its logical destination, and facing gradual dying might actually be a way for Americans to make their lives more peaceful. If our society can replace its technological panic over death with courage and empathy, if it can turn conflicts into friendships, it might enable a shift toward greater compassion.

· · ·

THE THIRD LESSON CAME in the final days of Betty Goyette. She had stopped taking food and water eight days previously; eternity was close at hand. Her husband, Art, heard that I fooled with the guitar some, and he asked me to come play for Betty. I could not possibly decline.

When I arrived Betty was aware that something was happening. Her room was crowded with Art and three of their five children, plus me and my instrument. They pursed their lips while I played simple classical pieces. Betty had not spoken in days, but her eyes were bright. I thought about various venues I had performed in my life—clubs, bars, coffeehouses, and theaters—and how unique this situation was. Then we agreed I should play one more before going. I thought about it a minute, about what song to leave her with, what last music. I played "Somewhere Over the Rainbow."

The room grew very quiet. I watched Betty, the lifelong choir member. She was screwing up one side of her face, making an O with her mouth, thrusting forward her chin. Her daughter Anne said, "My God, I think Mom is trying to sing."

Lesson three is that helping someone who is dying, even if just by providing brief entertainment, is one of the most gratifying experiences imaginable. No response from an audience will equal the gesture of a dying woman who heard me play an old song and wanted to join the tune.

As with my story about Geoff, the lesson goes well beyond my experience. It may even be universal, if you consider the story of Angola.

The Louisiana State Penitentiary at Angola is an eighteen-thousand-acre concentration of people who committed horrible crimes. One of the world's largest maximum-security prisons, it is filled to the gills because of Louisiana's arguably toughest-in-the-nation sentencing laws. Half of the five thousand inmates are serving life sentences. Prison hygiene being what it is, infectious diseases being the opportunists they are, about 85 percent of the inmates in Angola will die there.

Many inmates' first experience with death occurred when they committed murder. What restitution could there be for such an unforgivable deed? What possible remedy?

If there is any answer to these questions, it may be found in the Angola Prison Hospice. Just as in the real world, when people are irreversibly dying in a jail, it costs less and improves the quality of the patient's remaining life when hospice principles are applied.

The remarkable thing about Angola is not that it has a hospice unit; many prisons do. It is not even unusual to have inmates participate in a capacity similar to volunteers in the outside world. What is noteworthy is the effect that caring for the dying has on these criminals.

"I've seen guys that used to run around Angola, and want to fight and drug up, actually cry and be heartbroken over the patient," one inmate said in an Open Society Institute documentary about Angola. Prisoners slowly shed their hardened shells as they provide calm and tender care to dying friends and strangers, and as they see the fate that awaits all mankind.

"It's been very touching," another inmate said. "It's brought tears to my eyes, because you get in a relationship with the guys and it really hurts you. Being there for them, it takes a lot out of you. But it puts a lot in you."

A lot of what? The inmates don't ever say, exactly. But their tone and manner hints at something entirely new in their life. Convict volunteers care for dying buddies, help them achieve whatever peace they can with the demons they carry, provide intimate final services that range from praying to feeding to diapering, and eventually lower the bodies in plain coffins into graves on the prison grounds. And as they do this work, these criminals turn not toward God necessarily but toward meaning, toward the understanding that life has meaning, that their own life as damaged as it is might have value in its remaining days or months or years in prison.

Prison officials insist that the program is not about coddling criminals. The goal is to humanize the prison atmosphere, quite frankly to save some money, and to turn prisoners' time behind bars into something constructive.

A third inmate said that the hospice work has ended his overwhelming lifelong anger, making room for other emotions.

"I did a lot of wrong," he admitted. "I hurt a lot of people out there. When I heard about hospice, it was in my heart to join. Because I said, 'This will be my way of giving back to society. To tell people that I was sorry for what I did.'"

Lesson three is the same whether the caretaker is one of the worst members of society or simply a loving family member steadfast at the bedside. Caring for the dying is not a burden. It is a means to redemption.

If they can do it in Angola, they can do it in Peoria. The gratification of helping people at the end of their lives is within everyone's grasp.

THE FOURTH AND FINAL LESSON is the lesson of the leaves. In fall's bright colors nature makes it clear: The most important time in your life is not the moment of your death but the time as it approaches.

Dozens of people taught me that same lesson during my research. They did not fear death, but they feared dying badly. They did not want to live forever, but they wanted to live well for as long as possible. They did not want to die one moment too soon, but they did not want to suffer one moment too long. They all had goals for their remaining days, projects and conversations and holidays and family occasions—just like everyone else.

We are all in the same boat. We are all, each one of us, always proceeding toward the end that is inevitable. Each year we blithely pass the anniversary of our death, little acknowledging how much life is simply a journey toward that day. So, just like all those terminal patients, we are shaping the quality of our dying right this instant. If we want a meaningful death, then we must strive to live a meaningful life. Our days are numbered; the potential quality of our days is infinite.

The surest way to enrich that quality, and magnify its meaning, is to live a life mindful of its temporariness. As I interviewed people from all kinds of backgrounds, in all regions of the country, I saw how mortality helped them change priorities. Anyone would shift if told he or she had only a fixed amount of time to live. The reality, of course, is that everyone has a fixed amount of time. That could be a cause for fear, or it could have the opposite effect. Perhaps each day becomes more precious when we acknowledge that we have a limited supply of them.

That is the instruction from the leaves: The art of dying well is the art of living well. There is no telling when the story will finish. And so the most important time in your life is none other than right now.

SOURCES AND RESOURCES

GENERAL NOTES

Unless otherwise indicated, individuals' directly quoted comments came from interviews conducted in person or by phone, or in rare instances by e-mail. Whenever this was not the case, the source text or film is cited.

This book avoids the use of the term *doctor* when introducing an individual so as not to cause confusion between M.D.s and Ph.D.s, but subsequent references occasionally use *Dr.* to describe a physician.

One challenge when working with medical data is timeliness. The information here is the most current available. The exception is when two numbers are juxtaposed for purposes of comparison. In those instances the data used is for the most recent year in which both pieces of information are available. For example, a 1998 tally of hospitals is compared only with a 1998 tally of ICU beds, even if a 2001 count of hospitals is available.

INTRODUCTION

xi   Arlene Charron   The narrative relies on case documents obtained from the Vermont Medical Practice Board through the Freedom of Information Act and the Vermont Public Records Law. Further details were obtained during interviews with Vermont regulators and law-enforcement personnel, records at the Vermont Department of Health, and death certificate filings in the town of St. Johnsbury.

xiii   Norcuron   Information about the drug's uses came from Howard Shapiro, M.D. Information about morphine dosages and timing came from Zail Berry, M.D. Specifics about the uses, contraindications, and effects of Norcuron were drawn from the *Physicians' Desk Reference* and Joseph Nasca, M.D.

PART ONE: THE IMPRINT A BODY MAKES

3   Last Hours   Jack is a composite character, based on national average data from 1976 and today. A composite was necessary in order to portray an individual capable of dying twice, in two different ways. Every other individual in this book is an actual person identified by name, age, location, medical status, etc.

7   causes of death   Data drawn from the *National Vital Statistics Report,* a publication of the Centers for Disease Control and Prevention, and from the Web site of the National Center for Health Statistics. Several years' publications provided material, generally in the charts on death rates for selected causes. The data concerned 1972–92. For the subsequent ten years, the

information was supplemented by data for selected causes of death provided by the American Heart Association and the American Stroke Association. This source was confirmed and supported by "Preliminary Data for 2003," 53 *National Vital Statistics Report* 15 (Feb. 28, 2005). The incidence of heart disease and stroke remain high because the nation's population has grown, but the trends in rates of death from those causes have been consistently downward. For example, the number of deaths from heart disease dropped 9.9 percent from 1992 to 2002, but the rate of deaths from heart disease in that period fell 26.5 percent.

8   death from chronic respiratory disease   "Preliminary Data for 2003," 53 *National Vital Statistics Report* 15 (Feb. 28, 2005). The period of increase mentioned here was from 1979 to 1994.

8   Alzheimer's disease   Ibid., supplemented by information on the current number of people with the illness provided by the American Alzheimer's Association. The estimate of future cases came from Ed Edelson's December 15, 2005 report in *HealthDay*.

8   death rate from AIDS   Data from the HIV/AIDS Prevention Division at the Centers for Disease Control. The period under study was 1987–2000.

8   cancer   Data from the National Cancer Institute and the American Cancer Society. The 2005 statistical compilation of the American Heart Association also provided information.

8   evolution of human diet   Joe Friel, "Fuel," in *The Triathlete's Training Bible—Second Edition* (Boulder, Colo.: Velo Press, 2004), whose source was *The Paleo Diet For Athletes* by Loren Cordain, Ph.D. (Emmaus, Pa.: Rodale, 2005).

10   where people die   The Rand Institute study *Living Well at the End of Life,* by Joanne Lynn, M.D., M.A., M.S., and David Adamson. Additionally, the publication *New Study of Death Patterns in the United States* provides 1980s data from the National Mortality Followback Survey. That study, issued February 23, 1998, came from the National Center for Health Statistics.

14   EMTs   Data from the National Registry of Emergency Medical Technicians and *EMS Magazine.*

14   biological details of heart attacks and strokes   Interviews with physicians, and Sherwin Nuland, M.D., *How We Die* (New York: Knopf, 1994). That book also contributed to the description of a defibrillator's effect.

15   heart attack treatment protocols and quality measurements   Information from the Center for Medicare and Medicaid Services, a division of the federal Department of Health and Human Services.

15   number of heart-disease procedures and survival rates   "Heart Disease and Stroke Statistics—2005 Update" and "Open Heart Surgery Statistics," American Heart Association Web site.

16   stroke death rates and survival data   Ibid., Andrew Murr, "To Save the Stricken Brain," *Newsweek,* Dec. 8, 2003.

16   congressional safety acts   Norman Finkelstein, *The Way Things Never Were* (New York: Atheneum, 1999).

16–17   death rates due to accidents   National Center for Health Statistics Web site and "Preliminary Data for 2003," op. cit. The rate of deaths due to injury in the workplace also comes from these sources.

17   life expectancy   "Life Expectancy Hits Record High," *National Vital Statistics Report,* Feb. 28. 2005. The report, based on data from 2003, found life expectancies for white males at 75.4 years, black males at 69.2 years, white females at 80.5 years, and black females at 76.1 years. Each is a record high. Supplemental material about life expectancy came from *Living Well at the End of Life,* op. cit.

24   medical bills and bankruptcy   A joint study by Harvard Law School and Harvard Medical School of 1,771 personal-bankruptcy filings in five federal courts, as well as 931 follow-up telephone interviews with the filers. The study, written by David Himmelstein, Elizabeth Warren, Deborah Thorne, and Steffie Wollhandler, appeared in the February 2, 2005, issue of *Health Affairs.*

24   ICU patients' untreated pain   The $28 million "Study to Understand Prognoses and Preferences for Outcomes and Risks of Treatment" (hereinafter "SUPPORT project study") is considered definitive because it surveyed 9,105 seriously ill patients in detail, including following about half of the group until death. Numerous subsequent studies stemmed from SUPPORT's findings. Data about people spending their savings on dying patients' hospital care, about hospital patients' pain experiences, and about spending time on ventilators also come from the SUPPORT project.

24   ICU deaths after withdrawing life support   Nicholas Smedira, M.D., "Withholding and Withdrawal of Life Support from the Critically Ill," *New England Journal of Medicine* (Feb. 1990).

24   disregard for advance directives   SUPPORT project study.

24   However, only a fraction   The study on physicians failing to find out whether dying patients wanted to be resuscitated was conducted by the National Institute of Mental Health through the Robert Wood Johnson Foundation.

25–26   nursing homes   Research by several scholars at the John A. Hartford Center of Geriatric Nursing Excellence at the University of California at San Francisco, which in turn relied upon individual facility data made public by the federal Centers for Medicare and Medicaid Services. The percentages reflect the situation in 2003. The primary source for that information and for comparisons with past findings was Charlene Harrington, Helen Carillo, and Cassandra Crawford, *Nursing Facilities—Staffing, Residents and Facility Deficiencies 1997–2003.*

26   people's unwillingness to live in nursing homes   Thomas Mattimore, M.D., "Surrogate and Physician Understanding of Patients' Preferences for Living Permanently in a Nursing Home," *Journal of the American Geriatrics Society* (July 2001): 45:7.

26   percentage of Americans dying in nursing homes   Geriatrician Allen Ramsey, M.D.

26   congressional investigation   The Special Investigations Division of the U.S. House of Representatives Committee on Government Reform's "Abuse of Residents Is a Major Problem in U.S. Nursing Homes" tallied state inspections of the facilities between January 1, 1999, and January 1, 2000. The report became a public document on July 30, 2001.

26   "It would have been intolerable"   CBS News reported the comments of Congressman Henry Waxman of California on July 31, 2001.

27   National Association of Attorneys General   Interview with the NAAG's 2003 president, Drew Edmondsen of Oklahoma.

27   number of intensive-care beds   Interviews with officials at the American Hospital Association, as well as several editions of the book *Hospital Statistics,* published by Health Forum LLC, an affiliate of the AHA.

27   35,000 people in persistent vegetative state   Up to 25,000 adults and 10,000 children in a persistent vegetative state, "Medical Aspects of the Persistent Vegetative State" by the Multi-Society Task Force on PVS, *The New England Journal of Medicine* (May 1994).

29   "fragmented care system"   *Living Well at the End of Life,* op. cit.

29   Christine Cassel   *Approaching Death,* 1997 Institute of Medicine report, a definitive analysis of the status of care for people who are dying and a clearinghouse of pertinent research findings, is cited numerous times in this book. Thus, it merits fuller description. The institute is a thirty-five-year-old division of the National Academy of Sciences in Washington, D.C. The institute functions as an advisor to the federal government but also performs research on its own behalf. *Approaching Death* was approved by the governing board of the National Research Council, whose membership is the National Academy of Sciences, the National Academy of Engineering, and the Institute of Medicine. Marilyn Field, Ph.D., directed the study. The Committee on Care at the End of Life consisted of Christine Cassel, M.D., Robert Burt, J.D., Margaret Campbell, M.S.N., Robert Kliegman, M.D., Matthew Loscalzo, M.S.W., Joanne Lynn, M.D., M.A., M.S., Neil Macdonald, M.D., Willard Manning, Ph.D., Donald Patrick, Ph.D., Richard Payne, M.D., George Thibault, M.D., and Theresa Varner, M.S.W., M.A.

29   American Medical Association policy comments   *The Good Care of the Dying Patient* (AMA, 1996).

29   measurements of the quality of hospice   Ibid., which was produced by the AMA's Council on Scientific Affairs. These positions were summarized in *At Death's Door* by Michael deCourcy Hinds, a 1997 publication of the National Issues Forums Institute in Washington, D.C.

30   Karen Ann Quinlan   Marilynn Webb, *The Good Death* (New York: Bantam, 1997). This book also told the story of Karen's father's death.

30   Oregon's physician-assisted suicide rates   "The Seventh Annual Report on Oregon's Death with Dignity Act" issued March 10, 2005, by the Oregon Department of Human Services.

40   rate of hospice growth   According to Stephen Connor, Ph.D., Vice President for Research and International Development at the National Hospice and Palliative Care Organization, in 1996 the United States had 2,722 licensed provider sites for hospice care, serving approximately 450,000 patients. In 2000 there were 3,100 sites, which served 700,000 patients.

40   hospice utilization and length of stay   Barry Yeoman, "Going Home," *AARP Magazine* (Jan./Feb. 2005).

44   Wennberg   Dr. John Wennberg at Dartmouth Medical School has made a distinguished career of studying Medicare utilization. Chapter six of the *Dartmouth Atlas of Health Care* focuses on end-of-life care. Wennberg has also published papers and given talks on the lack of any demonstrable connection between spending on end-of-life care and the quality of care patients receive.

PART TWO: NOT AN EMERGENCY

53   "families bore the bulk of medical expenses"   *Living Well at the End of Life,* op. cit.

56   level of function/time figures   Many sources contributed to the graphs of illness trajectories, including physician interviews and the Rand paper, but the definitive source was the Institute of Medicine's book *Approaching Death.*

60   What happens when a person dies?   Discussion of the physical and emotional stages of dying relied on clinician interviews, as well as documents from the Hospice of Northeast Florida in Jacksonville. Many hospice organizations provide brochures with similar information to people who are dying and to their families. Nuland's *How We Die* again was influential.

62   "Interactions just like this"   Ira Byock, M.D., *Dying Well* (New York: Riverhead Books, 1997).

62   conflicts resulting from good intentions   Roeline Pasman, Ph.D., has performed several projects researching nursing home dilemmas. Her remarks here came from a 2004 collection of her papers, "Forgoing Artificial Nutrition and Hydration in Nursing Home Patients with Dementia."

63   Pasman's findings echo those reported in many U.S. medical journals   The practice of food and water cessation by terminal patients remains controversial within the medical community. Therefore, the assertions here are based on numerous sources: Linda Ganzini, M.P.H., Elizabeth Goy, Ph.D., Lois Miller, Ph.D., R.N., Theresa Harvath, R.N. Ph.D., Ann Jackson, M.B.A., and Molly Delorit, B.A., "Nurses' Experiences with Hospice Patients Who Refuse Food and Fluids to Hasten Death," 349 *New England Journal of Medicine* 4 (July 24, 2003); Franklin Miller, Ph.D., and Diane Meier, M.D., "Voluntary Death: A Comparison of Terminal Dehydration and Physician-Assisted Suicide," 128 *Annals of Internal Medicine* 7 (April 1, 1998); Timothy Quill, M.D., and Ira Byock, M.D., "Responding to Intractable Suffering: The Role of Terminal Sedation and Voluntary Refusal of Food and Fluids," 132 *Annals of Internal Medicine* 5 (July 3, 2000); C. J. Meares, Ph.D., R.N., "Primary Caregiver Perceptions of Intake Cessation in Patients Who Are Terminally Ill," *Oncology Nursing Forum* (Nov./Dec. 1997); L. A. Printz, "Terminal Dehydration: A Compassionate Treatment," 24:10 *Archives of Internal Medicine* (1992).

65   Elisabeth Kübler-Ross   She published many books on psychological issues at the end of life. *On Death and Dying* (New York: Macmillan, 1969) is generally regarded as her masterwork.

66   Julia story   Maggie Callanan and Patricia Kelley, *Final Gifts* (New York: Poseidon Press, 1992).

67 "We are just beginning to appreciate hope's reach" Jerome Groopman, M.D., *The Anatomy of Hope* (New York: Random House, 2004).

70 Mysteries of Life The mysteries of patient behavior at the end of life have been widely chronicled, including comprehensive research by Kübler-Ross and others. In *Final Gifts* Callanan and Kelley term these phenomena "near death awareness."

PART THREE: HEAL THYSELF

77 Doctors' Beginnings The history and process of academic dissection was obtained from interviews with medical students and anatomy professors, the photographic book *Anatomy of Anatomy* by Meryl Levin (Brooklyn: Third Rail Press, 2000), and "Anatomy Lessons: A Vanishing Rite for Young Doctors," March 23, 2004, by Abigail Zuger in *The New York Times*.

79 "Students are mandated to carry out" Kathy Johnson Neely, M.D., of Northwestern Memorial Hospice and Northwestern University Medical School, and Douglas Reifler, M.D., of Northwestern University Medical School, cowrote "Early Encounters with Death: Narrative Reflections of the First Year Medical Students."

82 "Textbooks serve as the cornerstone" Michael Rabow, M.D., Grace Hardie, M.D., Joan Fair, Ph.D., and Stephen McPhee, M.D., "Content of 50 Textbooks from Multiple Specialties," *Journal of the American Medical Association* (Feb. 9, 2000).

83 "Helpful information was rare" Annette Carron, D.O., Joanne Lynn, M.D., M.A., M.S., and Patrick Kearney, "End-of-Life Care in Medical Textbooks," *Annals of Internal Medicine* (Jan. 5, 1999).

84 analysis of fifty nursing textbooks Betty Ferrell, Ph.D., F.A.A.N., Rose Virani, R.N.C., B.S.N.N., M.H.A., O.C.N., and Marcia Grant, D.N.Sc., F.A.A.N., "Analysis of Symptom Assessment and Management Content in Nursing Textbooks," 2 *Journal of Palliative Medicine* 2 (1999).

84 "nurses and physicians cannot do what they do not know" Michael Rabow, Stephen McPhee, Joan Fair, and Grace Hardie, "A Failing Grade for End-of-Life Content in Textbooks: What Is to Be Done?" 2 *Journal of Palliative Medicine* 2 (1999).

85 Fourth-year medical students survey Heather Fraser, M.D., Jean Kutner, M.D., M.S.P.H., and Mark Pfeifer, M.D., "Senior Medical Students' Perceptions of the Adequacy of Education on End-of-Life Issues," 4 *Journal of Palliative Medicine* 3 (2001).

85 "Graduating medical students are inadequately trained" William Nelson, Ph.D., Nancy Angoff, M.D., Ellen Binder, M.D., Molly Cooke, M.D., Janet Fleetwood, Ph.D., Sarah Goodlin, M.D., Kenneth Goodman, Ph.D., Karen Orloff Kaplan, Sc.D., Thomas McCormick, D.Min., Mary Meyer, Miles Sheehan, M.D., Tom Townsend, M.D., Peter Williams, Ph.D., J.D., and William Winslade, Ph.D., J.D., "Goals and Strategies for Teaching Death and Dying in Medical Schools," 3 *Journal of Palliative Medicine* 1 (2000).

86 position of the Association of American Medical Colleges *Contemporary Issues in Medical Education* vol. 2, no. 1 (April 1999). Officials at the AAMC did not respond to numerous requests for interviews.

86 "dying is too important" *Approaching Death*, op. cit.

88 Montefiore Medical Center Study Charles Schwartz, M.D., Joseph Goulet, M.S., M.Phil., Victoria Gorski, M.D., and Peter Selwyn, M.D., M.P.H., "Medical Residents' Perceptions of End-of-Life Care Training in a Large Urban Hospital," 6 *Journal of Palliative Medicine* 1 (2003).

89 internal-medicine residency programs survey Patricia Mullan, Ph.D., David Weissman, M.D., Bruce Ambuel, Ph.D., and Charles Von Gunten, M.D., Ph.D., "End-of-Life Care in Internal Medicine Residency Programs: An Interinstitutional Study," 5 *Journal of Palliative Medicine* 4 (2002).

90 "My first year as an intern" Colin Murray Parkes, M.D., a bereavement psychologist and author in Great Britain, is quoted from his remarks in the 2003 film *Pioneers of Hospice*,

which was produced by Terrence Youk and the Madison-Deane Initiative, a program founded by two doctors' widows to increase public awareness of hospice.

91   Balfour Mount   From *Pioneers of Hospice*.

92   Robert Kane   Some of the narrative originated with Dr. Kane's personal statement on the Web site of Professionals with Personal Experience in Chronic Care. The rest came from a September 14, 2004, National Public Radio report on the organization by Joseph Shapiro.

93   "It is incumbent on the physician"   Timothy Quill, M.D., and Penelope Townsend, R.N., B.S.N., "Bad News: Delivery, Dialogue and Dilemmas," 151 *Archives of Internal Medicine* (March 1991).

98   Northwestern University study   "Early Encounters with Death," op. cit.

99   Thomas Jefferson University survey   Terri Maxwell, R.N., M.S.N., Emilie Passow, Ph.D., James Plumb, M.D., and Randa Sifri, M.D., "Experience with Hospice: Reflections from Third-Year Medical Students," 5 *Journal of Palliative Medicine* 5 (2002).

101   twenty-seven new interns   James Hallenbeck, M.D., and Merlynn Bergen, Ph.D., "A Medical Resident Inpatient Hospice Rotation: Experiences with Dying and Subsequent Changes in Attitudes and Knowledge," 2 *Journal of Palliative Medicine* 2 (1999).

103   Northwestern University's hospice intensive   Charles Von Gunten, M.D., Ph.D., Jeanne Martinez, R.N., M.P.H., Kathy Neely, M.D., Martha Twaddle, M.D., and Michael Preodor, M.D., "Clinical Experience in Hospice and Palliative Medicine," 1 *Journal of Palliative Medicine* 3 (1998).

108   Cleveland Clinic's palliative fellowship   J. Andrew Billings, M.D., "Palliative Medicine Fellowship Programs in the United States," 3 *Journal of Palliative Medicine* 4 (2000).

108   more than one million doctors   A definitive tally of the number of practicing physicians in America is not available because some doctors maintain licenses even though they are retired and some have licenses in several states. The Federation of State Medical Boards' annual report on doctor discipline in 2004 included state-by-state licensing counts, which totalled 1,048,090.

110   NIH conclusions   The National Institutes of Health held a three-day State of the Science conference on improving end-of-life care, December 6–8, 2004, which produced the policy statement quoted here.

111   "None of the faculty"   Eugenia Siegler, M.D., F.A.C.P., "The Rise and Fall of a Palliative Care Program at a Community Hospital," *Innovations in End-of-Life Care* (Feb. 2002).

112   criminal prosecutors   The story of Frank Fisher, M.D., was drawn from multiple sources, including news accounts during and after the trial, analysis of the case by the Cato Institute, the Web site following the case maintained by Our Chronic Pain Mission, the anti-drug-war advocacy site DRC.net, and Radley Balko's September 23, 2004, commentary on FoxNews.com. Comments on the case by Sally Satel, M.D., came from "Doctors Behind Bars: Treating Pain Is Now Risky Business" October 19, 2004, *The New York Times*.

113   Texas triplicate-prescription-form law   Marilyn Webb, *The Good Death* (New York: Bantam, 1997), citing articles in *Texas Medicine* in February of 1992 and *Pain Digest* in 1991.

113   AMA's formal policy on pain management   "About the AMA Position on Pain Management Using Opioid Analgesics," a policy statement from the Continuing Medical Education Division.

114   DEA-AMA collaboration   Sally Satel, M.D., *The New York Times*, Oct. 19, 2004; American Medical Association Web site; Mark Ingebretsen, "Doctors Concerned by Removal of DEA Pain-Medication Prescribing Guidelines," *MedPage Today*, Dec. 30, 2004.

115   "An oncologist who is uncomfortable with dying"   Anthony Back, M.D., "Oncology and Palliative Care: Are Oncologists Evil, or Just Oblivious?" 3 *Journal of Palliative Medicine* 1 (2000).

117   physicians showing grief   The exchange of letters between Bernard Siegel, M.D., and Stephen Schultz, M.D., appeared in 272 *Journal of the American Medical Association* 9 (Sept. 7, 1994).

118–119   Massachusetts General Hospital survey   Timothy Ferris, M.D., M.Phil., M.P.H., J. Anne Hallward, M.D., Larry Ronan, M.D., and J. Andrew Billings, M.D., "When the Patient Dies: A Survey of Medical House Staff about Care After Death," 1 *Journal of Palliative Medicine* 3 (1998).

120   Dr. Wennberg's findings   John Wennberg, Elliott Fisher, Therese Stukel, Jonathan Skinner, Sandra Sharp, and Kristen Bronner, "Use of Hospitals, Physician Visits and Hospice Care during Last Six Months of Life among Cohorts Loyal to Highly Respected Hospitals in the United States," 328 *British Medical Journal* (March 2004).

PART FOUR: MEDICINE AND LOVE ARE NOT THE SAME THING

127   John and Eiko Williams   Numerous newspaper reports about the incident when it occurred.

131–132   Duke University study   Catherine Breen, M.D., M.P.H., Amy Abernathy, M.D., Katherine Abbott, B.A., and James Tulsky, M.D., "Conflict Associated with Decisions to Limit Life-Sustaining Treatment in Intensive Care Units," 16 *Journal of General Internal Medicine* (May 2001).

132   study of end-of-life care based on setting   Joan Teno, M.D., M.S., Brian Clarridge, Ph.D., Virginia Casey, Ph.D., M.P.H., Lisa Welch, M.A., Terrie Wetle, Ph.D., Renee Shield, Ph.D., and Vincent Mor, Ph.D., "Family Perspectives on End-of-Life Care at the Last Place of Care," 291 *Journal of the American Medical Association* 1, (Jan. 7, 2004).

133   families viewed as "problems"   Carol Levine, M.A, and Connie Zuckerman, J.D., "The Trouble with Families: Toward an Ethic of Accommodation," 30 *Annals of Internal Medicine* (1999).

133–134   "emotional difficulties for . . . family and friends"   *Final Gifts*, op. cit.

138   number of Americans who move annually   2000 U.S. Census and a government analysis of the reasons that people moved, *Geographical Mobility*, by Jason Schachter, U.S. Census Bureau, August 2003.

143   survey of patients and their families   Ezekiel Emanuel, M.D., Ph.D., Diane Fairclough, D.P.H., Julia Slutsman, B.A., and Linda Emanuel, M.D., Ph.D., "Understanding Economic and Other Burdens of Terminal Illness: The Experience of Patients and Their Caregivers," 132 *Annals of Internal Medicine* 6 (March 2000).

144   Oregon study   Sylvia McSkimming, R.N., Ph.D., Marian Hodges, M.D., M.P.H., Alicia Super, R.N., B.S.N., Marie Driever, R.N., Ph.D., Mary Schoessler, R.N., Ed.D., Stephen Franey, M.A., and Melinda Lee, M.D., "The Experience of Life-Threatening Illness: Patients' and Their Loved Ones' Perspectives," 2 *Journal of Palliative Medicine* 2 (1999).

148   New York City study   Joel Cantor, Sc.D., Jan Blusten, M.D., Ph.D., Mathew Carlson, Ph.D., and David Gould, Ph.D., "Next-of-Kin Perceptions of Physician Responsiveness to Symptoms of Hospitalized Patients Near Death" 6 *Journal of Palliative Medicine* 4 (2000).

152   Economics of Dying   A cogent summary of the financial issues in end-of-life care appeared in *Approaching Death*. That book is the source for the information about studies of the economic impact of hospice and Medicare spending on care of the dying, as well as the possible savings from the use of advance directives. Much of the discussion of the cost of end-of-life care stems from the compendium of research gathered and summarized in that book.

153   Harvard study of personal bankruptcies   *Health Affairs* (Feb. 2, 2005), op. cit. Additional information comes from the February 3, 2005, posting on consumeraffairs.com.

154   Virginia Commonwealth University Medical Center study   The work of team leaders Tom Smith, M.D., and Patrick Coyne has been the subject of numerous articles in medical and general interest publications. The numbers used here come from Gautam Naik, "Unlikely Way to Cut Hospital Costs: Comfort the Dying," *The Wall Street Journal*, March 10, 2004.

156–57   Massachusetts General Hospital study   J. Andrew Billings, M.D., and Ellen

Kolton, B.A., "Family Satisfaction and Bereavement Care Following Death in the Hospital," 2 *Journal of Palliative Medicine* 1 (1999).

158 correlation between end-of-life care and family members' subsequent illnesses Geoffrey Cowley, Claudia Kalb, Anne Underwood, and Karen Springen, "Health for Life: Your Family & Your Health," *Newsweek*, April 25, 2005.

172–73 family members' view of their loved ones' care Joanne Lynn, M.D., M.A., M.S., Joan Teno, M.D., M.S., Russell Phillips, M.D., Albert Wu, M.D., M.P.H., Norman Desbiens, M.D., Joan Harrold, M.D., M.P.H., Michael T. Claessens, M.D., Neil Wenger, M.D., M.P.H., Barbara Kreling, B.A., and Alfred Connors Jr., M.D., "Perceptions by Family Members of the Dying Experience of Older and Seriously Ill Patients," 126 *Annals of Internal Medicine* 2 (Jan. 15, 1997).

PART FIVE: SMELLING THE ROSES

183–84 advance directives *Approaching Death,* op. cit. The book's conclusions stem from the SUPPORT study, among others.

184 reasons for Oregon physician-assisted suicides Annual reports on the Death with Dignity Act by the Oregon Department of Human Services.

000 kind of care patients with various terminal illnesses may predictably need J. Randall Curtis, M.D., M.P.H., F.C.C.P., Marjorie Wenrich, M.P.H., Jan Carline, Ph.D., Sarah Shannon, Ph.D., R.N., Donna Ambrozy, Ph.D., and Paul Ramsey, M.D., "Patients' Perspectives on Physician Skill in End-of-Life Care," 122 *Chest* (2002).

185 "ongoing ambivalence about power and control" Perspective piece by Timothy Gilligan, M.D., and Thomas Raffin, M.D., 125 *Annals of Internal Medicine* 2 (July 1996).

187 Weissman David Weissman, M.D., "Who is in Control?" 5 *Journal of Palliative Medicine* 1 (2002). Dr. Weissman is the publication's founding editor.

187–88 Oregon study Maria Silveira, M.D., M.A., Albert DiPiero, M.D., M.P.H., Martha Gerrity, M.D., Ph.D., and Chris Feudtner, M.D., M.P.H., Ph.D., "Patients' Knowledge of Options at the End of Life—Ignorance in the Face of Death," 284 *Journal of the American Medical Association* 19 (Nov. 15, 2000).

188 resuscitation survey SUPPORT project study, op. cit.

197 Carole Gaudreault maintained her mobility for six months following this interview, spent about three months with diminishing movement in her legs, and died at home on Valentine's Day 2006.

201 Lorraine Barstow Interviews with her son John, supplemented by his unpublished writings on the topic.

208 CPR survival rates on television shows Susan Diem, M.D., M.P.H., John Lantos, M.D., and James Tulsky, M.D., "Cardiopulmonary Resuscitation on Television: Miracles and Misinformation," *New England Journal of Medicine* 334: no. 24 (June 13, 1996). The CPR survival rates on British TV shows is 30 percent, according to Anthony Mazzarelli, a graduate student in law, bioethics, and medicine at the University of Pennsylvania, who wrote on this topic in the October 5, 2001, issue of bioethics.net.

209 DNR study Daniel Sulmasy, O.F.M., M.D., Ph.D., and Jessica McIlvane, Ph.D., "Patients' Ratings of Quality and Satisfaction with Care at the End of Life," 162 *Archives of Internal Medicine* (Oct. 14, 2002).

210–211 wishes of people who are dying Joanne Lynn, M.D., M.A., M.S, and Joan Harrold, M.D., *Handbook for Mortals* (New York: Oxford University Press, 1999); David Kessler, *The Needs of the Dying* (New York: HarperPerennial, 2000); and particularly Eric Cassell, M.D., *The Nature of Suffering* (New York: Oxford University Press, 2004). Further information came from Peter Singer, M.D., M.P.H., Douglas Martin, Ph.D., and Merrijoy Kelner, Ph.D., "Quality End-of-Life Care—Patients' Perspectives," 281 *Journal of the American Medical Association* 2 (Jan.

13, 1999); Laurel Herbst, M.D., Joanne Lynn, M.D., M.A., M.S., Alan Mermann, M.D., M.Div., and Jill Rhymes, M.D., "What Do Dying Patients Want and Need?" *Patient Care* (Feb. 28, 1995).

211 "easier to get open heart surgery than Meals on Wheels" Joanne Lynn, M.D., "Travels in the Valley of the Shadow." This essay appeared in the book *Empathy and the Practice of Medicine: Beyond Pills and the Scalpel,* Howard Spiro et al., editor (New Haven, Conn.: Yale University, 1993).

211 "elevation of the science of medicine" Perspective piece by Gilligan and Raffin in the *Annals of Internal Medicine,* op. cit.

211–12 study of nonmedical issues Linda Emanuel, M.D., Ph.D., Hillel Alpert, Sc.M., B.Sc., DeWitt Baldwin Jr., M.D., and Ezekiel Emanuel, M.D., Ph.D., "What the Terminally Ill Care About: Toward a Validated Construct of Patients' Perspectives," 3 *Journal of Palliative Medicine* 4 (2000).

212 communication barriers between doctors and patients J. Randall Curtis, M.D., M.P.H., Donald Patrick, Ph.D., M.S.P.H., Ellen Caldwell, M.S., and Ann Collier, M.D., "Why Don't Patients and Physicians Talk about End-of-Life Care?" 160 *Archives of Internal Medicine* (June 12, 2000).

213–14 Brigham and Women's study Craig Lilly, M.D., Dawn De Meo, M.D., Larry Sonna, M.D., Ph.D., Kathleen Haley, M.D., Anthony Massaro, M.D., Robert Wallace, M.P.H., and Sean Cody, R.N., M.S.N., M.B.A., "An Intensive Communication Intervention for the Critically Ill," 109 *American Journal of Medicine* (Oct. 15, 2000).

214–15 Quill Timothy Quill, M.D., "Initiating End-of-Life Discussions with Seriously Ill Patients: Addressing the 'Elephant in the Room,'" 284 *Journal of the American Medical Association* 19 (Nov. 15, 2000).

216 Chalmers Roberts Chalmers Roberts experienced sudden heart failure on April 8, 2005. He died at home. He was ninety-four.

PART SEVEN: THE LESSON OF THE LEAVES

245 The source for any data or research in this section that is not cited below has already been identified in a prior chapter. For example, the Richmond, Virginia, study of money saved by providing inpatient hospice rather than regular hospital care is cited in the notes to Part Four.

249 Open Society Institute and Robert Wood Johnson Foundation funding David McGrew, M.D., "Funders Leaving the Field," 6 *Journal of Palliative Medicine* 4 (2003).

250 estimating death within six months Joanne Lynn, M.D., M.A., M.S., *Sick to Death and Not Going to Take It Anymore!* (Berkeley: University of California Press, 2004).

251 83 percent of Americans currently dying are covered by Medicare That percentage is often cited; one source is David Introcaso, Ph.D., and Joanne Lynn, M.D., M.A., M.S., "Systems of Care: Future Reform," 5 *Journal of Palliative Medicine* 2 (2002).

252–54 Paul Bilder Board of Medical Examiners, State of Oregon, stipulated order of April 17, 2003; complaint and notice of proposed disciplinary action of August 12, 2002; stipulated order of Sept. 1, 1999; complaint and notice of proposed disciplinary action of March 19, 1999.

254 policy implications of end-of-life care Jaya Rao, M.D., M.H.S., Lynda Anderson, Ph.D., and Suzanne Smith, M.D., M.P.H., M.P.A., "End of Life Is a Public Health Issue," 23 *American Journal of Preventive Medicine* 3 (2002).

256 Henry James Ben Rich, J.D., Ph.D., "Prioritizing Pain Management in Patient Care," 110 *Postgraduate Medicine,* no. 3 (Sept. 2001).

256 Wing Chin Ibid., supplemented by Matthew Yi's report in the *San Francisco Chronicle* on June 14, 2001, and information at the law center of CNN.com.

258–59   medical centers' initiatives to improve end-of-life care   Joanne Lynn, M.D., Janice Lynch Schuster, and Andrea Kabcenell, R.N., M.P.H., *Improving Care for the End of Life, a Sourcebook for Health Care Managers and Clinicians* (New York: Oxford University Press, 2000).

259   Joint Commission on Accreditation of Healthcare Organizations   Carol Curtiss, M.S.N., R.N., *Orthopedic Nursing* (March 1, 2001).

260   demographic limitations to establishing nationwide hospice   Data from the Hospice of Connecticut.

260   St. John's Regional Medical Center study   *The Case for Hospital-Based Palliative Care*, published by the Center to Advance Palliative Care. Gains in care management and other aspects of palliative medicine came from the same publication.

260   "Medicine evolved throughout the centuries"   Mary Bretscher, M.D., and Edward Creagan, M.D., "Understanding Suffering: What Palliative Medicine Teaches Us," 72 *Mayo Clinical Procedures* (August 1997).

262–64   "Serendipitous ripples"   Pippa Hall, B.Sc., M.D., C.C.F.P., M.Ed., "Serendipitous Ripples: Unexpected Outcomes of a Palliative Care Educational Project," 4 *Journal of Palliative Medicine* 3 (2001).

267   Committee on Bioethical Issues   Jeffrey Berger, M.D., Fred Rosner, M.D., Joel Mpotash, M.D., Pieter Kark, M.D., and Allen Bennett, M.D., "Communication in Caring for Terminally Ill Patients," 3 *Journal of Palliative Medicine* 1 (2000).

267   UCLA researchers   Kenneth Rosenfeld, M.D., Neil Wenger, M.D., M.P.H., and Marjorie Kagawa-Singer, Ph.D., "End-of-Life Decision Making, a Qualitative Study of Elderly Individuals," 15 *Journal of General Internal Medicine* (Sept. 2000).

268   Reverend Donald Moore   A professor of theology at Fordham University in New York City, he is quoted January 16, 2005, *The New York Times*.

273–74   Angola   The documentary *Angola Prison Hospice* was produced by the Open Society Institute with funding from the Soros Foundation.

OTHER RESOURCES

The following books and films also contributed to this work, either forming, sustaining, or challenging my point of view. They are listed in alphabetical order by primary author, editor, or producer.

Armstrong, Lance. *It's Not About the Bike: My Journey Back to Life*. New York: Putnam, 2000.

Bayley, John. *Elegy for Iris*. New York: St. Martin's Press, 1999.

Brown, Chip. *Good Morning Midnight: Life and Death in the Wild*. New York: Riverhead, 2003.

Byock, Ira. *Dying Well*. New York: Riverhead, 1997.

Callanan, Maggie, and Patricia Kelley. *Final Gifts*. New York: Poseidon Press, 1992.

Carlson, Lisa. *Caring for Your Own Dead*. Hinesburg, Vt.: Upper Access, 1987.

Cassell, Eric. *The Nature of Suffering and the Goals of Medicine*. New York: Oxford University Press, 1991.

Davis, F. A., ed. *Taber's Cyclopedic Medical Dictionary*.

Estess, Jenifer, as told to Valerie Estess. *Tales from the Bed: On Living, Dying and Having It All*. New York: Atria Books, 2004.

Finkelstein, Norman H. *The Way Things Never Were*. New York: Atheneum, 1999.

Gerson, Michael. *The Second Brain*. New York: HarperCollins, 1998.

Gerteis, Margaret, Susan Egdman-Levitan, Jennifer Daley, and Thomas Delbanco, eds. *Through the Patient's Eyes*. San Francisco: Jossey-Bass, 1993.

Gladwell, Malcolm. *The Tipping Point*. Boston: Little, Brown, 2000.

Groopman, Jerome. *The Anatomy of Hope: How People Prevail in the Face of Illness*. New York: Random House, 2004.

Harrington, Charlene, Helen Carillo, and Cassandra Crawford. *Nursing Facilities—Staffing, Residents and Facility Deficiencies 1997–2003.*

Hogan, Cornelius, Deborah Richter, and Terry Doran *At the Crossroads*, privately published, 2005.

Kessler, David. *The Needs of the Dying*. New York: HarperPerennial, 2000.

Kübler-Ross, Elisabeth. *On Death and Dying*. New York: Macmillan, 1969.

Lakoff, George. *Don't Think of an Elephant*. White River Junction, Vt.: Chelsea Green, 2004.

Levin, Meryl. *Anatomy of Anatomy*. Brooklyn: Third Rail Press, 2000.

Levine, Stephen. *Who Dies?* Garden City, N.Y.: Doubleday, 1982.

Lynn, Joanne, and Joan Harrold. *Handbook for Mortals: Guidance for People Facing Serious Illness*. New York: Oxford University Press, 1999.

Lynn, Joanne, Janice Lynch Schuster, and Andrea Kabcenell. *Improving Care for the End of Life: A Sourcebook for Health Care Managers and Clinicians*. New York: Oxford University Press, 2000.

McKibben, Bill. *Enough: Staying Human in an Engineered Age*. New York: Times Books, 2003.

The Merck Manual of Medical Information, 1997 ed., home edition.

Moyers, Bill, producer. *On Our Own Terms*. Documentary series produced for public television, 2000.

Nuland, Sherwin. *How We Die*. New York: Knopf, 1994.

Parkes, Colin Murray, Pittu Laungani, and Bill Young, eds. *Death and Bereavement across Cultures*. New York: Routledge, 1997.

Pasman, Roeline. *Forgoing Artificial Nutrition and Hydration in Nursing Home Patients with Dementia*. Institute for Research in Extramural Medicine, Netherlands Ministry of Health, Welfare and Sports, 2004.

Roberts, Chalmers M. *How Did I Get Here So Fast?* New York: Warner, 1991.

Rosenfeld, Arthur. *The Truth About Chronic Pain*. New York: Basic Books, 2003.

Ryerson, Marjorie. *Companions for the Passage: Stories of the Intimate Privilege of Accompanying the Dying*. Ann Arbor: University of Michigan Press, 2005.

Sacks, Oliver. *The Man Who Mistook His Wife for a Hat and Other Clinical Tales*. New York: Summit Books, 1985.

Shames, Laurence, and Peter Barton. *Not Fade Away*. Emmaus, Pa.: Rodale, 2003.

Sogyal, Rinpoche. *The Tibetan Book of Living and Dying*. Rev ed. San Francisco: HarperSanFrancisco, 2002.

Webb, Marilyn. *The Good Death: The New American Search to Reshape the End of Life*. New York: Bantam, 1997.

Williams, Marjorie. *The Woman at the Washington Zoo*. New York: Public Affairs, 2005.

Youk, Terrence, producer. *Pioneers of Hospice*. Film produced for the Madison-Deane Initiative to improve end-of-life care.

INTERNET SOURCES

Centers for Disease Control's National Center for Health Statistics: www.cdc.gov/nchs/hus.htm

American Medical Association: www.ama-assn.org

American Nurses Association: www.nursingworld.org

American Hospital Association: www.hospitalconnect.com

Growth House, a comprehensive clearinghouse and source of links for hospice and home-care resources and issues: www.growthhouse.org

Americans for Better Care of the Dying: www.abcd-caring.org

National Hospice and Palliative Care Organization: www.nhpco.org

American Hospice Foundation: www.americanhospice.org

American Cancer Society: www.cancer.org

Last Acts (the former Robert Wood Johnson Foundation program to improve end-of-life care): www.lastacts.org

Open Society Institute (the former program to improve public awareness about end-of-life-care options and successes): www.soros.org

American Heart Association: www.americanheart.org

American Stroke Association: www.strokeassociation.org

Alzheimer's Association: www.alz.org

ALS Association (Lou Gehrig's disease): www.alsa.org

National Multiple Sclerosis Society: www.nmss.org

International Association for Organ Donation: www.iaod.org

ACKNOWLEDGMENTS

This book disproves the conventional belief that writing is a solitary act. Throughout, I relied on an army of researchers, doctors, patients, lobbyists, theologians, nurses, policy wonks, loved ones of people who had died, writers, family, and friends. Not a word is mine alone.

My foremost thanks go to Arthur Goyette, whose courage and faith extended not only to his wife, Betty, but also to a stranger he entrusted with the privilege of witnessing her remarkable last months. While teaching me what was possible, Art became a good friend. Caroline Crawford connected me with YoungWidow.org, a national resource for young widows and widowers through which I met many people with great stories to tell. I regret that more of them did not make it into this book. I am also indebted to the other families and patients who allowed me to ask them such intimate questions at such painful moments. I prize their courage.

Big thanks are due, too, to people who aided the medical research. Dr. Terry Rabinowitz connected me with interRAI, an international group, in the effort to establish objective measurements for the quality of medical care. Mike Noble at Fletcher Allen Health Care was a great help at introducing me to end-of-life care experts. Frank McDougall, a trusted friend, gave me an excellent tutorial on the workings of Medicare, and linked me with medical sages within Dartmouth-Hitchcock Medical Center. For early exposure to hospice, I am grateful to Dawn Stanyon and Angel Collins of the Visiting Nurse Association of Chittenden and Grand Isle Counties, and Sharon Kregan of the Respite House. Dr. Rosemary Johnson-Hurzeler at the Connecticut Hospice generously opened her facility's doors to me. Dr. Zail Berry saved me weeks of research by permitting me to plunder her medical library. With comments on an early draft,

Zail also rescued me from many clinical errors. Any that remain are my fault.

A number of people facilitated this book with advice, suggestions, even places to stay during research travel: Luke Albee, Beth Donovan, Jym Wilson, and Donelle Blubaugh. Thanks go to Geoff Gevalt, for urging me to chase the story about Dr. Tim Thompson. Gratitude goes to Justin Cronin as well, for concluding a long phone call with the observation that the subject about which I could not stop talking might make for a book. Carolyn Edwards, Ph.D., was a wise and essential guide. My friend Dave Wolk helped me find early audiences for these ideas, and offered timely moral support during the research.

Several people read early drafts, or listened when I read sections aloud, and their counsel has been invaluable: Candace Page, Dana Yeaton, Deborah Porter, Ph.D., and Mark Nash. From this work's conception to publication, I benefited from the faith and friendship of Michelle Everleth. Foremost in this group, however, is my brother Dr. Mike Kiernan, whose integrity is so great he overcame objections to portions of this book, then made incisive suggestions for its improvement. I further beg the indulgence of all my siblings for what is an admittedly partial rendering of our parents' deaths.

In 2003, Linda Loewenthal interrupted a family vacation to take a cell phone to the beach and listen for an hour while I outlined the idea for this book. It was only the beginning of her helpful and attentive work as my agent and friend. A writer could not ask for a better guide and advocate. Fortuitously, she introduced me to George Witte at St. Martin's, who instantly understood the project and believed in it. George's later editing suggestions honed the book immeasurably, and his team at St. Martin's astonished me with their engagement and enthusiasm. I feel fortunate to have been in such capable hands.

Above all, from start to finish, I have benefited from the advice, support, and friendship of Chris Bohjalian—which is far more than literary. Chris has been patient beyond belief and generous beyond my deserving.

This project has been a humbling and moving education. To all who taught me so much, I am grateful.

INDEX

American Medical Association (AMA)
  assisted suicide position by, 30,
    262
  EPEC program by, 104–5, 108
  pain management policies by, 113–14,
    115
  unwarranted care findings by, 29
American Society of Clinical Oncology,
    115
Americans for Better Care of the Dying,
    153, 211, 266
aneurysms, 223–25, 271
Angell, Kenneth, xiii
anger stage (death), 65–67
Annals of Internal Medicine, 133, 173,
    186
  humanity issues addressed in, 211
Approaching Death study, 29, 279n29
  medical training findings in, 85
Archives of Internal Medicine, 84
Artists Who Care, 36
assisted suicide. *See* physician-assisted
    suicide
Association of American Medical
    Colleges (AAMC), 86
autopsies, 119

Back, Anthony, 115
bankruptcy, 24, 153, 266
bargaining stage (death), 65–67
Barstow, John, 201–3
Barstow, Lorraine, case study
  illness in, 201
  post-death care in, 201–3
Barstow, Richard, 201, 203
Beauchamp, Ann, 134–37
Beauchamp, Bob, case study
  health-care system issues in, 135–37
  illness in, 134–35
Bengston, Paul, xi, xiii
bereavement services, 258–59
  doctors' responsibilities regarding,
    119, 158
  hospice provision of, 172
Bergman, William, 256
Berry, Zail, 95–98, 105
Bilder, Paul, 252–54
Billings, Andrew, xiv
Brigham and Women's Hospital,
    Massachusetts, 213
Brodeur, Susan Goyette, 160–71. *See
    also* Goyette, Betty, case study
Brooklyn Hospital Center, New York, 111

Burlington Free Press, xii
Bush, George W., 248, 257
Byock, Ira, 61–62, 86–87, 107–8

California, legislation in, 252
Callahan, Bob, 233–38
Callanan, Maggie, 66, 133
calling a code, 207–9
Canada, palliative care in, 91, 104,
    262–64
cancer, xv, 13, 115, 116
  case studies featuring, 96–97,
    160–75, 179–82, 188, 194–97,
    199–206, 233–39, 273
  doctors' rotations and, 88
  occurrence statistics for, 8
  trajectory of, 56–57
cardiopulmonary resuscitation (CPR),
    46, 215
  media portrayal of, 208, 284n208
  training for, 14, 266
Carron, Annette, 83
case studies, palliative care
  Alexander, 199–201
  Barstow, 201–3
  Charron, ix–xiv, xviii
  Gaudreault, 195–97
  Goyette, 160–75, 273
  Grace, 96–97
  Hanley, 194
  "Jack," 18–22, 277n3
  Jakubek, 203–6
  Kiernan, Mary, 233–41
  Waller, 197–99
case studies, traditional health-care
  Beauchamp, 134–37
  Cross, 179–82, 188
  "Jack," 3–6, 277n3
  Kiernan, Peter, 223–32
  Meenan, 145–51
  Schuyler, 139–43
  Stannus, 130–31
  Waller, 197–99
Cassel, Christine, 29
Center for Evaluative Clinical Sciences
    at Dartmouth, New Hampshire, 44
Center to Advance Palliative Care, 43
Charron, Arlene, case study
  disciplinary action in, xviii
  drug administration in, xi
  illness in, ix–x
  medical controversy in, xi–xiv
  ventilator withdrawal in, x–xi